Health Seeking Behavior and Out-of-pocket Expenditure on Chronic Non-communicable Diseases in Sub-Saharan Africa

Challenges
in Public Health

Editor: Prof. Dr. Oliver Razum, Bielefeld

Formerly/früher: Medizin in Entwicklungsländern
Herausgegeben von
Prof. Dr. Hans Jochen Diesfeld, Heidelberg

Volume 66

*Zu Qualitätssicherung und Peer Review
der vorliegenden Publikation*

Die Qualität der in dieser Reihe
erscheinenden Arbeiten wird
vor der Publikation durch den
Herausgeber der Reihe geprüft.

*Notes on the quality assurance
and peer review of this publication*

Prior to publication, the
quality of the work published
in this series is reviewed
by the editor of the series.

Qun Wang

Health Seeking Behavior and Out-of-pocket Expenditure on Chronic Non-communicable Diseases in Sub-Saharan Africa

The Case of Rural Malawi

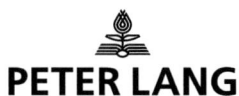

PETER LANG

Bibliographic Information published by the Deutsche Nationalbibliothek
The Deutsche Nationalbibliothek lists this publication in the Deutsche
Nationalbibliografie; detailed bibliographic data is available in the internet
at http://dnb.d-nb.de.

Library of Congress Cataloging-in-Publication Data
A CIP catalog record for this book has been applied for
at the Library of Congress.

Thanks to Dalian University of Technology as the
sponsor of this book (grant number: DUT16RC(3)041).

ISSN 1863-768X
ISBN 978-3-631-71739-4 (Print)
E-ISBN 978-3-631-74118-4 (E-PDF)
E-ISBN 978-3-631-74119-1 (EPUB)
E-ISBN 978-3-631-74120-7 (MOBI)
DOI 10.3726/b12995

© Peter Lang GmbH
Internationaler Verlag der Wissenschaften
Berlin 2018
All rights reserved.

Peter Lang – Berlin · Bern · Bruxelles · New York ·
Oxford · Warszawa · Wien

This publication has been peer reviewed.
www.peterlang.com

To my parents,
For always encouraging me to fulfill my dreams

To my colleagues and friends in Heidelberg,
For giving me the best memory in my life

Acknowledgements

This book is based on the dissertation which I completed as a requirement for obtaining my doctoral degree. The three years of the PhD study was the best time in my life. I really have to thank a lot of people. Without them, I would have never been able to do so.

First and foremost, I need to thank PD. Dr. Manuela De Allegri, my supervisor, from the bottom of my heart. She taught and showed me the whole process of doing research and trained me from a person who loves research to becoming a real scientist. All the documents full of her comments witness how often and how much she guided me, which are my greatest treasure and which I have reserved very well and will reserve forever.

My sincere gratitude also goes to Prof. Dr. med. Rainer Sauerborn. It is him who gave me an opportunity of becoming a PhD student in this well-known institute and cared about my progress whenever we met. For setting foot in Heidelberg, I have to thank Prof. Dr. Hengjin Dong, who recommended me to Prof. Dr. med. Rainer Sauerborn. Whenever I visited his home in Heidelberg, I felt like I was in my home country.

I need to express my special thanks to Dr.med. MPH Stephan Brenner. He supported me all the time during my PhD study and gave me many influential suggestions on how to conduct my research.

Thanks to the financial support of my government, I was able to do my research without worry. I will dedicate my life to making my home country different.

Many thanks to Olivier Kalmus, Alex Z. Fu, Julia Lohmann, and Gerald Leppert for their support during my data analysis. I am grateful for Christabel Kaminjolo-Kambala, Jacob Mazalale, Kassim Kwalamasa, and Hastings Thomas Banda for their great support in helping me quickly understand everything about Malawi. I also need to thank Rasul Fatema for her help in proofreading my thesis.

A special thanks to Dr. Aurelia Souares for her organization of several workshops on NCD, which really broadened my mind. Another key source of energy for my thesis is from Gilbert Abiiro, Nguyen Hoa Thi, Wulifan Joseph, Albino Kalolo, Lara Gautier. We shared lots of good memories and I will cherish their friendship forever. Great support for my thesis also comes from Dr. Revati Phalkey, Yan Ding, Dr. Paulina Grys, Dr. Peter Dambach, Dr. Andreas Deckert, Dr. Budi Aji, and Dr. Shafiu Mohammed. They finished their PhD study earlier than me and shared with me a lot of experience in both academic research and life in Heidelberg.

Many thanks to the administrative support from Angela Haefner, Laura Di Lorenzo, and Sandra Niebel, they really helped me through many difficulties.

Last but not least, I must thank my parents for their high expectation which is always the biggest motivation for me to progress. During these years, I am very happy to see that my husband and I really learned to understand and support each other and work together to make our future life better even though we are a bit far away.

Table of Contents

Abbreviations

CNCDs	Chronic non-communicable diseases
NCDs	Non-communicable diseases
WHO	World Health Organization
CVDs	Cardiovascular diseases
SSA	Sub-Saharan Africa
USD	United States Dollars
LMICs	Low- and middle- income countries
HICs	High-income countries
SES	Social-economic status
OOP	Out-of-pocket
COI	Cost-of-illness
Int$	international dollars
KES	Kenia-Schilling
TZS	Tanzania-Schilling
NGN	Nigerian Naira
ZAR	South African Rand
GDP	Gross Domestic Product
MoH	Ministry of Health
MoLGRD	Ministry of Local Government and Rural Development
CHAM	Christian Health Association of Malawi
BLM	Banja La Mtsogolo
EHP	Essential Health Package
SLAs	Service Level Agreements
SACCO	Bvumbwe Savings and Credit Cooperative
REACH Trust	Research for Equity and Community Health Trust
MNL	Multinomial logit model
iid	Independently and identically distributed
IIA	Independence of irrelevant alternatives

CL	Conditional logit model
NL	Nested logit model
OLS	Ordinary least square
GLM	Generalized linear model
EEE	Extended estimating equations
MWK	Malawian Kwacha
SD	Standard deviation
MHI	Micro health insurance

List of Tables

List of Figures

1. Introduction

1.1 Chronic non-communicable diseases (CNCDs)

1.1.1 Definition of CNCDs

CNCDs are responsible for the largest portion of the global burden of disease (World Health Organization, 2005). Literally, CNCDs are closely related to chronic diseases and non-communicable diseases (NCDs).

Chronic diseases include numerous and diverse conditions with the vast majority of them being incurable. They have no single, universally accepted medical definition because numerous differences exist among various chronic diseases in terms of the causes, course, changeability and consequences (Zeidner and Endler, 1995). Nowadays, the World Health Organization (WHO) uses common features that various chronic diseases share to define chronic diseases: they last long, usually gradually progress, and need systematic and long-term approaches for treatment (World Health Organization, 2005). While in population-based surveys the working definition of chronic diseases varies across different studies, studies from the United States of America (U.S.), Kenya, and Burkina Faso defined chronic diseases as those diseases that had lasted for longer than three months (Gans, 1988; Su *et al.*, 2006a; Chuma *et al.*, 2007). One study from South Africa considered chronic diseases as conditions that had persisted for longer than four weeks (Goudge *et al.*, 2009a). Another study on chronic diseases from Southern India viewed respondents had suffered from chronic diseases if they had taken medications consecutively for at least 30 days (Bhojani *et al.*, 2013). In addition, in a different study from India, any condition that had lasted more than three weeks and required long-time management was defined as chronic diseases (Mondal *et al.*, 2010).

It has also aroused considerable debates in recent studies about what is a NCD (Sridhar *et al.*, 2011). The answer seems straightforward. However, the only shared component across definitions of NCDs is that they comprise conditions that are not transmissible between people. Even within the same organization, NCDs are defined differently in various contexts and for diverse purposes. In the website of the WHO, NCDs are referred to as those conditions known as chronic diseases and not transferable from person to person (World Health Organization, 2014a). This simple definition can be easily understood and accepted by the lay people. NCDs are not equal to chronic diseases since some chronic diseases are caused by infectious agents, like HIV/AIDS, tuberculosis. From the view of the global disease burden, the WHO defines NCDs differently, including diseases and conditions ranging from cardiovascular diseases (CVDs), cancers, chronic respiratory diseases, and diabetes to visual and hearing impairment and mental illness (World Health Organization, 2008a). While in the recent publications on global status and policy guidelines to prevent and control NCDs by the WHO, NCDs have been narrowed down to cover only four major health conditions: CVDs, cancers, chronic respiratory diseases, and diabetes since these conditions share common modifiable risk factors, i.e. tobacco use, physical inactivity, unhealthy diet, and harmful use of alcohol, and thus have common methods to prevent and control them (World Health Organization, 2008b, 2011a). This narrow definition of NCDs omits other conditions like blindness and mental health, which also needs continued care.

This study focused on how people cope when they chronically suffer from non-infectious conditions. I adopted a broader scope of NCDs and used the terminology of CNCDs to represent the broader definition of NCDs, which is in line with previous studies (Yang *et al.*, 2008; Schmidt *et al.*, 2011). CNCDs are defined as diseases or conditions that affect individuals over an extensive period of time. In contrast to communicable illnesses, CNCDs are rarely caused by the transmission of infectious agents, but are predominantly the result of longstanding exposure to a single or a combination of risk factors (Daar *et al.*, 2007).

1.1.2 CNCDs worldwide

Currently, CNCDs are the leading cause of death in all World Bank regions except Sub-Saharan Africa (SSA) (Figure 1.1) (World Health Organization, 2008c). In 2005, out of about 58 million deaths worldwide, 35 million (60%) were caused by CNCDs (World Health Organization, 2005). Globally, the leading causes of deaths related to CNCDs are CVDs (30% of all deaths), cancers (13%), chronic respiratory diseases (7%), and diabetes (2%) (World Health Organization, 2005). In addition, the WHO predicted that deaths due to CNCDs will rise by 15% worldwide (to about 44 million) between 2010 and 2020. The region of Africa has been predicted to witness the greatest increase (27%) of deaths attributable to CNCDs, followed by the region of South-East Asia and the Eastern Mediterranean. While the region of Europe was predicted to see no increase of CNCDs deaths during this period (World Health Organization, 2008b).

Beyond the disease burden, CNCDs also pose a considerable financial burden, since treating CNCDs, once expressed clinically, is very expensive due to a much longer time of care than treating acute communicable diseases (Suhrcke et al., 2006). Globally, the financial burden due to CNCDs has been projected to be 3.6 trillion United States Dollars (USD) in 2010 and 6.7 trillion USD by 2030 (Bloom et al., 2011).

Figure 1.1: Projected deaths (000s) by cause, in World Bank Regions in 2008.

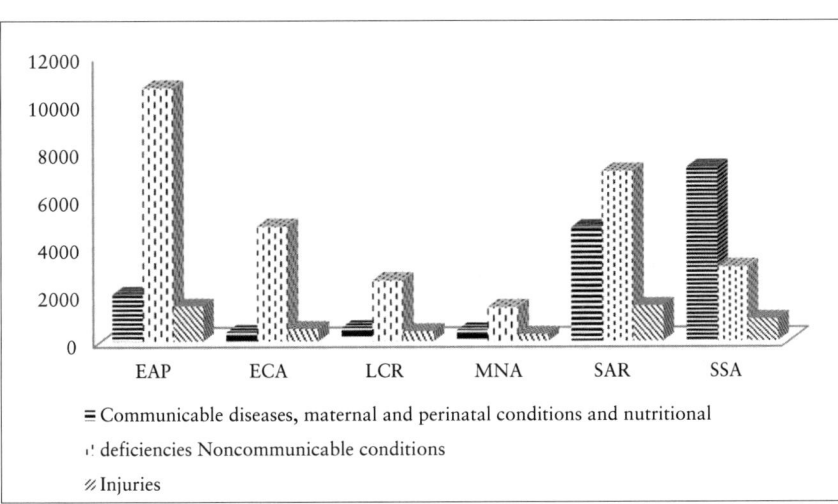

Notes: EAP = East Asia and Pacific; ECA = Europe and Central Asia; LCR = Latin America and Caribbean; MNA = Middle East and North Africa; SAR = South Asia; SSA = Sub-Saharan Africa.

Source: World Health Organization, 2008c.

1.1.3 CNCDs in low- and middle-income countries

Low- and middle- income countries (LMICs) are heavily affected, accounting for at least 80% of all deaths related to CNCDs (World Health Organization, 2005). In 2010, the overall age-standardized CNCD mortality rates in LMICs were 756 per 100 000 for males and 565 per 100 000 for females, which were respectively 65% and 85% higher than those for males and females in high-income countries (HICs). Till 2030, the WHO projects that CNCDs in LMICs will account for nearly five times as many deaths as communicable, maternal, perinatal, and nutritional conditions in these settings (World Health Organization, 2011a).

CNCDs have brought high financial burden to LMICs. It has been estimated that in 2010 alone, the economic loss due to CNCDs amounted to 500 billion USD in LMICs, accounting for 4% of these countries' GDP (WHO, 2011a). In spite of the fact that LMICs have far more population with CNCDs than HICs, at the time being HICs still pay much higher costs for CNCDs than LMICs. However, LMICs are projected to exceed HICs in terms of CNCDs costs by 2030, suggesting the high growth rate of financial burden due to CNCDs in LMICs by 2030 (Bloom *et al.*, 2011). Moreover, poverty and CNCDs are interconnected in LMICs. On one hand, the poor in LMICs are more likely to develop CNCDs and die prematurely (World Health Organization, 2005). On the other hand, CNCDs can easily lead the vulnerable population into deeper poverty in these settings (Engelgau *et al.*, 2012; Gotsadze *et al.*, 2009; Kankeu *et al.*, 2013; Rahman *et al.*, 2013; Sun *et al.*, 2009; Van Minh and Xuan Tran, 2012; World Health Organization, 2005; Su *et al.*, 2006a; Xu *et al.*, 2006b).

1.1.4 CNCDs in SSA

Even though communicable, maternal, perinatal, and nutritional conditions are still the leading cause of death in SSA, many countries in SSA face a rising CNCD 'epidemic' (Dalal *et al.*, 2011). In 2008, the WHO estimated 27.6% of all deaths in SSA to be caused by CNCDs, with a projected increase to 46.3% by 2030 (World Health Organization, 2008a). In 2010, the overall CNCD age-standardized death rates by sex in the region were already the highest in the world, 844 per 100 000 for males and 724 per 100 000 females (World Health Organization, 2011a).

What worsens the current situation in SSA is the wider age range of the people suffering from CNCDs and the higher prevalence of CNCDs among the very young population in SSA compared with other LMICs (Aït-Khaled *et al.*, 2001; Unwin *et al.*, 2001; Lopez *et al.*, 2006). This suggests an earlier onset of CNCDs and severer premature death caused by CNCDs in SSA (World Health Organization, 2011a, 2012). In 2008, out of all CNCDs deaths for males and females in SSA, 23% and 20% respectively occurred under the age of 45, while only 3% and 2% respectively were below the age of 45 in HICs (World Health Organization, 2008c). In SSA, the hard living environment, recurring infectious illnesses, and long-term stress for living aggregate the premature aging of body functioning, which may explain the earlier onset of CNCDs in the region (Miszkurka *et al.*, 2012). This special feature of the 'epidemic' of CNCDs in SSA negatively affects human productivity and socio-economic development in the region (Unwin *et al.*, 2001; World Health Organization, 2005).

1.1.5 The WHO and United Nations initiatives toward the four major health conditions and other CNCDs

In order to respond to the increasing disease burden due to the four major health conditions, over the past decade, the WHO has established global objectives and outlined proposed action plans for its member states, the Secretariat, and its international partners to prevent and control these conditions (World Health Organization, 2000, 2008b, 2008d, 2012) and related common risk factors (World Health Organization, 2003a, 2004a, 2010) (Figure 1.2). In addition, in 2011 the United Nations organized a high-level meeting to make an international commitment to fight against the four major health conditions, suggesting that they should be included in the global development agenda. This was the second time that General Assembly convened for a health issue; the first time was for HIV/AIDS (Figure 1.2) (United Nations General Assembly, 2011).

Especially in Africa, after analyzing current situations in the region, the WHO has issued regional strategies to guide its member states to address the emerging disease burden of CNCDs in these settings (Figure 1.3) (World Health Organization Regional Office for Africa, 2000a, 2000b, 2005, 2006, 2007, 2008, 2011; World Health Organization, 2003b). The diseases which the regional guidelines focus on are not only the four major health conditions worldwide, but also other common CNCDs in the region, such as sickle-cell diseases and oral health problems. To address the increasing disease burden of CNCDs, the health system in SSA needs to be restructured, which requires an initial understanding, currently lacking, of how communities currently cope with CNCDs (Dalal et al. 2011; Unwin 2001).

Figure 1.2: The WHO and United Nations initiatives towards the four major health conditions (CVDs, cancers, chronic respiratory diseases, and diabetes).

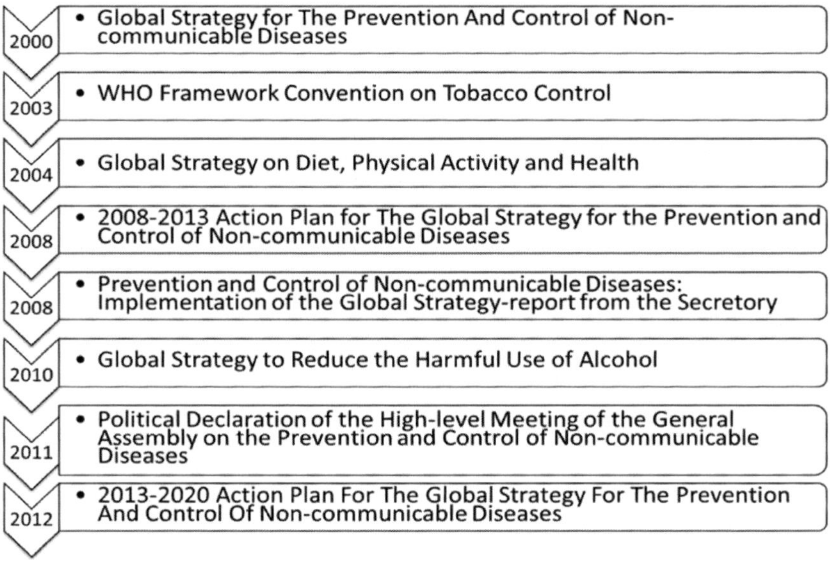

2000	• Global Strategy for The Prevention And Control of Non-communicable Diseases
2003	• WHO Framework Convention on Tobacco Control
2004	• Global Strategy on Diet, Physical Activity and Health
2008	• 2008-2013 Action Plan for The Global Strategy for the Prevention and Control of Non-communicable Diseases
2008	• Prevention and Control of Non-communicable Diseases: Implementation of the Global Strategy-report from the Secretory
2010	• Global Strategy to Reduce the Harmful Use of Alcohol
2011	• Political Declaration of the High-level Meeting of the General Assembly on the Prevention and Control of Non-communicable Diseases
2012	• 2013-2020 Action Plan For The Global Strategy For The Prevention And Control Of Non-communicable Diseases

Sources: World Health Organization, 2000, 2003, 2004a, 2008a, 2008b, 2010, 2012b; United Nations General Assembly, 2011.

Figure 1.3: The WHO initiatives towards CNCDs in Africa.

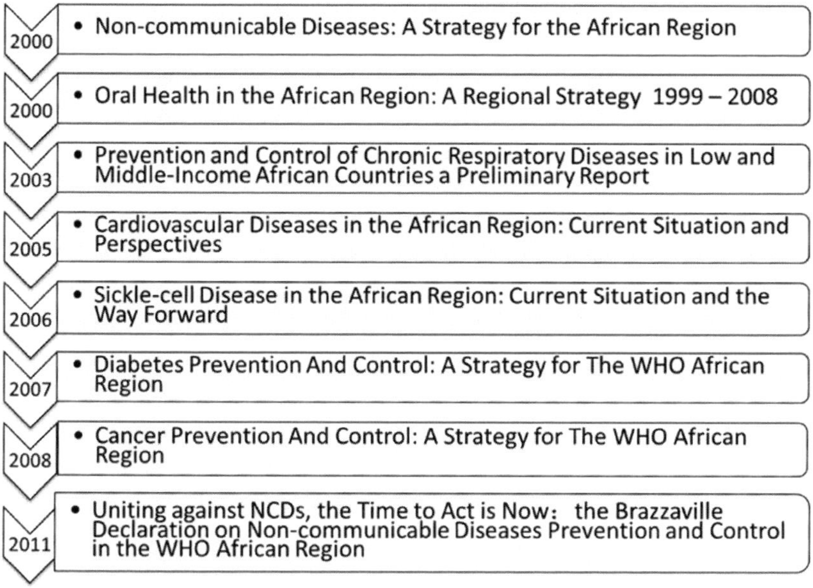

2000 • Non-communicable Diseases: A Strategy for the African Region

2000 • Oral Health in the African Region: A Regional Strategy 1999 – 2008

2003 • Prevention and Control of Chronic Respiratory Diseases in Low and Middle-Income African Countries a Preliminary Report

2005 • Cardiovascular Diseases in the African Region: Current Situation and Perspectives

2006 • Sickle-cell Disease in the African Region: Current Situation and the Way Forward

2007 • Diabetes Prevention And Control: A Strategy for The WHO African Region

2008 • Cancer Prevention And Control: A Strategy for The WHO African Region

2011 • Uniting against NCDs, the Time to Act is Now: the Brazzaville Declaration on Non-communicable Diseases Prevention and Control in the WHO African Region

Sources: World Health Organization Regional Office for Africa, 2000a, 2000b, 2005, 2006, 2007, 2008, 2011; World Health Organization, 2003a.

1.2 Health seeking behavior

Health seeking behavior refers to any activity undertaken by individuals who perceive themselves to have a health problem, to find an appropriate remedy (Kasl and Cobb, 1966). The concept of health seeking behavior needs to be interpreted carefully from that of health care seeking behavior. The concept of health seeking behavior centers on the 'process', i.e. the overall response starting from individual perceived illness, while the concept of health care seeking behavior centers on the 'end point', i.e. utilization of formal health care facilities (Tipping and Segall, 1995; MacKian, 2003). So the scope in the work related to health seeking behavior is wider than that related to health care seeking behavior (MacKian, 2003). The concept of health seeking behavior should also be differentiated from an even broader terminology – health behavior, which refers to any activity that healthy people take to prevent illnesses (Kasl and Cobb, 1966).

In SSA, compared with acute communicable diseases, researchers have paid less attention to studies on CNCDs. The majority of the scarce research available on CNCDs in SSA has focused on estimating disease or risk factor prevalence (Soliman and Juma, 2008; de Ramirez et al., 2010; Dalal et al., 2011; Msyamboza et al., 2011, 2012; Addo et al., 2012; Miszkurka et al., 2012; Phaswana-Mafuya et al., 2013), attributable mortality (Cooper et al., 1998; Bradshaw et al., 2007; Mayosi et al., 2009; Mbanya et al., 2010; Hall et al., 2011), and/or relevant treatment options (Cooper et al., 1998; Seedat, 2000; Beran and Yudkin, 2006; Azevedo and Alla, 2008; Mbanya et al., 2010). I could identify only six qualitative, 11 quantitative and three mixed methods studies on health seeking behavior for CNCDs in SSA. Hereafter these 20 studies are reviewed with a focus on two aspects 1) whether people use health services and in what facilities people choose to use services; 2) what factors influence their choices for health service utilization (MacKian, 2003).

1.2.1 Health seeking options on CNCDs in SSA

People who perceive themselves to be ill have the following health seeking options: no treatment, formal care (western care), use of traditional healers, and home treatment (self-medication). As for chronic diseases, whether people seek care on a continuous basis is also an important aspect for studies on care-seeking options.

In SSA, most of the limited evidence on CNCDs found that a considerable proportion of people with CNCDs do not seek any care in these settings. Using data from 870 households in Kenya, researchers found that more than 50% and 40% of those reporting chronic illnesses in rural and urban communities respectively did nothing for their chronic diseases (Chuma et al., 2007). Similarly, from a household survey on a sample of 1446 individuals in rural communities in South Africa, 48% of respondents reporting chronic diseases did not take any action for care (Goudge et al., 2009a). Among all the staff in a University in Nigeria, 29.4% of those reporting high blood pressure chose to do nothing for their condition (Faronbi et al., 2014).

Unlike the wide use of formal care in Western countries (MacKian, 2003), the use of formal care for CNCDs is relatively limited among community residents who report CNCDs in SSA. Out of 1102 middle-aged and older females in South Africa, about one third of those reporting CNCDs chose formal care (Lopes Ibanez-Gonzalez and Norris, 2013). Similarly, in an another community-based study in South Africa, 35% of those reporting chronic diseases sought formal care (Goudge *et al.*, 2009a). However, a few studies using data from patients with clear clinical diagnosis of CNCDs found that the utilization rate of formal care is relatively high. Out of 440 patients diagnosed with hypertension in South West Nigeria, more than 60% sought formal care (Osamor, 2011). A qualitative study in Uganda showed that all 24 respondents diagnosed with diabetes along with severe symptoms related to diabetes used formal care (Hjelm and Atwine, 2011).

Use of traditional care is another important source of treatment for CNCDs in SSA. A qualitative study from South Africa held the view that many people with cervical cancer used western and traditional care concurrently (Langley and Mary, 2012). In a qualitative study in Malawi, some respondents with cervical cancer were found to visit traditional healers first instead of going to formal facilities (Chadza, 2012). Out of 1365 hypertensive patients receiving care from five hospitals in Nigeria, 21% would turn to traditional care after the treatment in formal facilities (Oke and Bandele, 2004). A qualitative study from Uganda found that most of those who felt their treatment in the formal sector had failed decided to turn to traditional healers (Hjelm and Atwine, 2011).

In addition, home treatment has been observed to be a popular channel of health care for CNCDs. One quantitative study from Kenya found that 39.0% and 36.4% of respondents suffering from chronic diseases in the urban and rural settings respectively chose self-medication (Chuma *et al.*, 2007). Another quantitative study from Nigeria showed that people using self-medication accounted for 42.5% of those suffering from hypertension (Faronbi *et al.*, 2014).

Unlike acute conditions which require short-term care, CNCDs require continued care. However, in most areas in SSA continued care is often suboptimal (World Health Organization Regional Office for Africa, 2011). In a poor urban community in southwest Nigeria, out of 440 community residents diagnosed with hypertension, more than 40% had poor compliance with their long-term treatment. Once people felt better, they discontinued their treatment (Osamor and Owumi, 2011). Among 108 hypertensive patients from several facilities in a semi-urban community in Nigeria, only 33.3% adhered to their treatment even though more than 90% of all respondents had serious hypertension (Iyalomhe and Iyalomhe, 2010). However, in some least poor urban communities in SSA, people show better treatment compliance. Out of 192 patients diagnosed with diabetes from three public hospitals in urban South Africa, more than 90% sought care regularly and only less than 1% sought care only when necessary (Makinga and Beke, 2013).

1.2.2 Factors associated with health seeking behavior for CNCDs in SSA

1.2.2.1 Demand-side factors

Awareness, knowledge, beliefs, and perception of CNCDs

Out of the limited evidence on health seeking behavior on CNCDs in SSA, quite a few have reported very low awareness and knowledge on CNCDs among people in these settings (Kiawi et al., 2006; Iyalomhe and Iyalomhe, 2010; Birhanu et al., 2012), even among those patients with CNCDs at the very late stage of their conditions (Kidanto et al., 2002; Kazaura et al., 2007). The limited awareness and knowledge on CNCDs result in delays in seeking care for CNCDs in SSA (Kidanto et al., 2002; Kazaura et al., 2007; Chadza, 2012; Langley and Mary, 2012). In addition, a number of studies have reported that a very large proportion of people in SSA believed that CNCDs were caused by disrespectful spirits and unacceptable behaviors and thus they only trust traditional healers when seeking care (Kiawi et al., 2006; Iyalomhe and Iyalomhe, 2010; Birhanu et al., 2012; Chadza, 2012). Such belief and perception also brought stigma to people suffering from CNCDs, making them hesitant to reveal their conditions to the community, and thus chose home-based care (Birhanu et al., 2012). Beyond malevolent spirits and behavior, other studies also revealed that a considerable portion of people considered hypertension to be caused by poisoning and rotten food and mental stress (Iyalomhe and Iyalomhe, 2010), diabetes by excessive sugar consumption (Kidanto et al., 2002; Kiawi et al., 2006), and obesity to represent 'good living' in the region (Kiawi et al., 2006).

Financial resources

Lack of financial resources is one of the most important reasons for people not to seek any care for CNCDs (Goudge *et al.*, 2009a; Petricca *et al.*, 2009; Osamor and Owumi, 2011; Chadza, 2012). Having limited ability to pay is also a key factor for people with CNCDs to opt for informal care instead of formal care (Kiawi *et al.*, 2006; Osamor, 2011; Birhanu *et al.*, 2012).

Furthermore, among limited studies on health seeking behavior on CNCDs, quite a few found that the poorest seek less care than the least poor. A quantitative study in South Africa indicated that the wealthiest 30% of the population with high blood pressure used more than twice the amount of treatment than the poorest 40% (Alberts *et al.*, 2003). In another quantitative survey on a sample of 306 staff in one University in Nigeria, individuals from a higher social-economic status (SES) monitored their blood pressure much more often than those with a lower SES (Faronbi *et al.*, 2014). Another nation-wide quantitative study from South Africa found that the wealthiest used more medications for chronic conditions than the poor (Steyn and Levitt, 2006). In a qualitative study interviewing 29 diabetes patients, their family members, and related health workers, researchers found that the least poor had better access to diabetes-related drugs and treatment than the poor (Kolling *et al.*, 2010). Exceptionally, in a system which provides officially free services in government clinics in South Africa, SES was found not to influence health seeking behavior for chronic diseases (Goudge *et al.*, 2009a).

Proper health insurance coverage can help a person gain adequate access to health services. However, health insurance coverage is very limited across SSA (World Health Organization Regional Office for Africa, 2011). Only one quantitative study from South Africa addressed the role of health insurance in treatment seeking behavior for CNCDs and indicated that people with health insurance utilized more medications for chronic diseases than those without (Steyn and Levitt, 2006).

Perceived severity of diseases/stage of disease

In SSA, perceived severity of disease has long been reported as one of the primary factors determining health seeking behaviors in case of illness (Gotsadze *et al.*, 2005; Dong *et al.*, 2008). For CNCDs, perceived severity of disease is closely linked with stage of disease. When CNCDs are at an early stage, i.e. the best time to initiate control, people may have no or mild symptoms though pathologically CNCDs are already present. Thus, CNCDs at an early stage are usually not perceived to be severe by people. Once people perceive these conditions to be severe, these conditions are usually at a middle or late stage, when treating and controlling them becomes more complicated and expensive than that at an early stage (World Health Organization, 2011a, 2011b).

Researchers found that people in SSA either do not seek early treatment for chronic conditions, or choose informal care when their conditions are not perceived to be severe. In a mixed methods survey from South Africa, having a perceived mild condition was the main reason for nearly half of respondents not having sought any care for their chronic diseases (Goudge et al., 2009a). One qualitative study in Ethiopia found that the vast majority of respondents with cervical cancer preferred traditional care when their conditions were at an early stage (Birhanu et al., 2012). Meanwhile, researchers also found that people in SSA do not seek care for CNCDs until their conditions are at an advanced stage. In one qualitative study in Ethiopia, a great number of women with symptoms of cervical cancers only sought care when they were unable to tolerate the pain related to cervical cancer (Birhanu et al., 2012). Another qualitative study from Ethiopia found that people with rheumatic heart disease sought care when they suffered from symptoms related to the disease on a continuous basis (Petricca et al., 2009). In two quantitative surveys conducted in two teaching hospitals in Tanzania, 70% and 90% of their newly admitted cancer patients were at an advanced stage of the disease respectively (Kidanto et al., 2002; Kazaura et al., 2007).

Sex

Among the limited studies on health seeking behavior on CNCDs in SSA, only one study explicitly addressed the role of sex in health seeking behavior on CNCDs in these settings. The study found that in Uganda female diabetic patients sought follow-up treatment more often than male patients; while male patients were more often to choose private facilities than female patients. When the treatment in the formal sector failed, women were more likely to turn to traditional care than men (Hjelm and Atwine, 2011).

1.2.2.2 Supply-side factors

Health systems in SSA have long been structured to provide care for acute communicable and maternal conditions (Unwin *et al.*, 2001; Boutayeb and Boutayeb, 2005; Azevedo and Alla, 2008; Dalal *et al.*, 2011). Facing the emerging CNCDs, the health provision capacity for CNCDs in SSA has not been integrated into health systems and is generally lower compared with other regions of the world (World Health Organization Regional Office for Africa, 2011).

Availability of medications and services for CNCDs is very limited in SSA, especially at public hospitals, which deteriorates people's health and/ or discourages those with CNCDs from using health care, especially formal care. One qualitative study from Malawi found that when respondents with cervical cancer sought care at an early stage of the disease in the primary health care facilities, the staff there either gave them inappropriate drugs, or wrong diagnosis, or were simply absent from the facility. Thus they had to visit several health facilities before they finally got the right diagnosis and treatment, but at that time the disease had already become severe (Chadza, 2012). Another qualitative study in Ethiopia found that knowing the unavailability of diagnosis and treatment for cervical cancer, most affected women simply stayed at home without taking any actions (Birhanu *et al.*, 2012). Using qualitative data from diabetes patients in Tanzania, researchers found that many respondents with the disease usually sought care at private pharmacies because drugs were never available at public hospitals (Kolling *et al.*, 2010).

Accessibility of health care, defined in relation to the distance to health facilities as well as transportation possibilities (Abiiro *et al.*, 2014), is also decisive in influencing treatment seeking for CNCDs in SSA. One qualitative study from Malawi found that long distances deterred the majority of cervical cancer patients from utilizing care at an early stage at the primary health care facilities, in spite of the fact that services were available free of charge (Chadza, 2012). In a quantitative study in South Africa, researchers found that unaffordable transportation prevented people from accessing care at governmental clinics, even though it was officially free of charge (Lopes Ibanez-Gonzalez and Norris, 2013). In another qualitative study interviewing 33 rheumatic heart disease patients and caregivers in Ethiopia,

25 respondents disclosed that long distance and unaffordable transportation kept them from attaining follow-up treatment (Petricca *et al.*, 2009). Compared with western care, traditional care is found to be easier to access in SSA, which is another crucial reason for people to choose traditional care (Osamor, 2011; Birhanu *et al.*, 2012).

1.2.3 Knowledge gap in health seeking behavior on CNCDs in SSA

The available evidence on health seeking behavior on CNCDs in SSA mainly conveys the following information: 1) a large proportion of people with CNCDs in SSA do not seek care; 2) different sources of health care (including formal care, traditional care, and home care) for CNCDs coexist in SSA; 3) limited evidence is available on factors associated with health seeking choices for CNCDs in SSA; 4) out of all 20 reviewed studies, 16 focused on only one CNCD, three on chronic diseases with most of their cases suffering from HIV/AIDS (Steyn and Levitt, 2006; Chuma *et al.*, 2007; Goudge *et al.*, 2009a), and only one on a wide range of CNCDs (Lopes Ibanez-Gonzalez and Norris, 2013); 5) out of 11 reviewed quantitative studies, only two relied on population-based data with both of them being in South Africa (Steyn and Levitt, 2006; Lopes Ibanez-Gonzalez and Norris, 2013); 6) all of the reviewed quantitative studies exclusively used descriptive statistics and as such, they could not control for possible confounders (Kidanto *et al.*, 2002; Alberts *et al.*, 2003; Chuma *et al.*, 2007; Kazaura *et al.*, 2007; Iyalomhe and Iyalomhe, 2010; Langley and Mary, 2012; Lopes Ibanez-Gonzalez and Norris, 2013; Makinga and Beke, 2013; Faronbi *et al.*, 2014). Reflecting on the available evidence, one can conclude that there is urgent need for a quantitative study, more specifically looking at factors affecting treatment choices for CNCDs.

1.3 Out-of-pocket expenditure (OOP)

The World Bank defines OOP expenditure as any direct expenses paid by households, including tips and in-kind outlays, to health staff and providers of drugs, medical checks, or other goods and services, primarily used to restore or enhance individual or household members' health status (World Bank, 2014a). In spite of recent calls to advance the program towards universal health coverage, OOP payments are the principal means to finance health care in many LMICs (Gottret *et al.*, 2008). Transportation costs are included into the computation of OOP expenditure, since they depict the total cost of accessing health care (Gertler and Gaag, 1990).

The rapid spread of CNCDs in SSA bears an important burden to national health care systems, already strained in their capacity to provide coverage with quality services for maternal and acute conditions and to ensure adequate financial protection for their populations. Thus, much of the financial burden is shifted to local populations, who, in spite of already living at the margin of poverty, are asked to contribute directly towards the cost of care for CNCDs through direct OOP spending (Gottret and Schieber, 2006). Considering the paucity of adequate social protection structures in most SSA countries (WHO, 2011b), the increasing economic burden due to CNCDs is likely to become 'catastrophic' and aggravate poverty among local communities, who already struggle to meet basic daily needs (Goryakin and Suhrcke, 2014).

Given this increasing disease burden, understanding both the patterns of OOP spending as well as identifying sub-groups at specific risk of incurring high OOP spending for CNCDs, represent an essential step towards the development of adequate policies to protect those most at risk from facing impoverishment due to illness. However, as mentioned earlier, CNCDs have long been paid much less attention in SSA than acute communicable diseases and maternal care. The most relevant evidence on OOP expenditure on CNCDs comes from high-income countries (HICs) (Kankeu *et al.*, 2013). To date, there are very few studies that have addressed costs in relation to seeking care for CNCDs: 16 quantitative studies, one case study, and one mixed methods study.

1.3.1 Overall OOP expenditure on CNCDs and its breakdown in SSA

Among the 18 studies mentioned above, four studies specifically focused on OOP expenditure for CNCDs (Obi and Ozumba, 2008; Goudge *et al.*, 2009a; Huffman *et al.*, 2011; Gustafsson-Wright *et al.*, 2012), while the remaining 14 were cost-of-illness (COI) studies. Out of 14 COI studies, 12 reported the direct cost of CNCDs from the perspective of patients (Chale *et al.*, 1992; Pestana *et al.*, 1996; Neuhann *et al.*, 2002; Elrayah *et al.*, 2005; Aikins, 2007; Chuma *et al.*, 2007; Pepper *et al.*, 2007; Elrayah-Eliadarous *et al.*, 2010; Guinhouya *et al.*, 2010; Cavanagh *et al.*, 2012; Odili and Okwuanasor, 2012; Tagoe, 2013), while the remaining two used multi-country data and calculated the direct cost of CNCDs from the perspective of society (Kirigia *et al.*, 2009; Zhang *et al.*, 2010). Given that all these 18 studies have different study settings and disease categories, I do not intend to directly compare their numeric results. In spite of these differences, these 18 studies have all come to the same conclusion – the overall financial burden on CNCDs in SSA is already quite considerable. Based on the measure of financial burden and data source, these 18 studies can be classified into four groups as follows.

First, six out of 18 studies on overall OOP expenditure on CNCDs not only reported the absolute value of OOP expenditure, but also estimated the financial burden due to CNCDs borne by households by calculating the proportion of OOP expenditure on CNCDs to the annual/monthly household total income/expenditure. Based on 498 CVD patients receiving hospitalization care in Tanzania, researchers found the median for 15-month OOP expenditure for CVD care ranged from 374 international dollars (Int$) to 1137 Int$, which accounted for 7.1%-8.2% of the total annual household expenditures (Huffman *et al.*, 2011). Collecting data from 822 adult diabetes patients from clinics in Sudan, investigators estimated the annual direct cost per diabetic patient to be at 175 USD, which was equivalent to approximately 9% of the average annual earnings of these diabetes patients in the setting (Elrayah-Eliadarous *et al.*, 2010). One study from Nigeria found that out of 95 cervical cancer patients who were sent to radiotherapy treatment, only 19% took the treatment and all of them come from higher SES. The rest 81% did not receive the treatment because of financial difficulties. For those who could afford the treatment about 30% of their annual earnings were paid for radiotherapy (Obi and Ozumba, 2008). Obtaining data from 870 households from the community, one study from Kenya found that the mean direct cost per household for chronic diseases was 609 Kenia-Schilling (KES) in urban areas and 194 KES in rural areas, occupying respectively 5.7% and 5.0% of their household monthly expenses (Chuma *et al.*, 2007). Using data from 147 parents whose children were diagnosed with type 1 diabetes from facilities in urban Sudan, researchers found that the median annual direct cost per diabetic child was 283 USD, totaling 65% of their annual household expenditure on health and 23.2% of their annual household income (Elrayah *et al.*, 2005). One mixed methods study from South Africa found that OOP expenditure for repeated treatment for chronic diseases took up 6% to 60% of the household monthly income. The fluctuation depended upon the number of visits to health facilities and means of transportation (Goudge *et al.*, 2009a).

Meanwhile, another four studies estimated the financial burden from CNCDs by calculating the proportion of OOP expenditure on CNCDs to an objective measure (i.e. not varied by households), for instance, national minimum wage or the average income of certain subpopulations. Based on data from both hospitals and patients, researchers in Ghana found that the direct cost for insulin per patient per month was about 7 USD – 10 USD, totaling 40%-60% of monthly earnings of an average farmer in rural Ghana (Aikins, 2007). Similarly, collecting data from 412 stroke patients from one hospital in Togo, scientists found that the direct cost for stroke per patient was 680 Euro with an average of 17.4 hospitalization days, which was about 20 times as high as the minimum monthly income of a civil servant in the setting (Guinhouya *et al.*, 2010). Likewise, some researchers analyzed data from 474 diabetes patients in one hospital in Tanzania and found that the mean monthly direct cost for an insulin-dependent patient accounted for about one fourth of the national monthly minimal wage (Neuhann *et al.*, 2002). In one case study, researchers developed two hypothetical patients with diabetic foot ulcers and compared the direct cost of treating the two cases across several countries. They found that treating case one and case two cost 0.8 month and 24.8 months of the average monthly income in Tanzania respectively, while the cost equaled to 0.2 month and 9.6 months of the average monthly income in the US respectively (Cavanagh *et al.*, 2012).

Second, some studies reported the high financial burden of CNCDs by displaying the difference of the total OOP health expenditure between people with CNCDs and without, which is different from studies in the first group that only reported the OOP expenditure for CNCDs only. Using data from community members in Tanzania and Kenya, a study found that the average OOP expenditure for people with chronic diseases and those without was 2434 KES and 1565 KES respectively in Kenya, and 24880 Tanzania-Schilling (TZS) and 17111 TZS respectively in Tanzania

(Gustafsson-Wright *et al.*, 2012). Another survey from 4,124 households in Ghana found that the mean direct cost for households with at least one member reporting CNCDs was almost 50% higher than that for households without any member reporting CNCDs (Tagoe, 2013).

Third, a number of studies only depicted the absolute amount of financial burden for CNCDs in SSA without calculating the proportion of OOP expenditure for CNCDs to household expenditure. Using data from 40 diabetic inpatients in Nigeria, the mean direct cost per diabetic inpatient within an average duration of admission being 8.8 days was estimated at 15,600 Nigerian Naira (NGN) (Odili and Okwuanasor, 2012). Based on data from 53 hyperglycemic admissions to one hospital in South Africa, the mean direct cost per hyperglycemic admission was estimated at 5,309 South African Rand (ZAR), which was even more than the mean direct cost per HIV/AIDS admission (4,630 ZAR) in the same hospital at the same time (Pepper *et al.*, 2007).

Fourth, several studies used secondary data to estimate the financial burden of CNCDs at the national level, including a few based on multi-country data. One study from the WHO used data from 46 countries in Africa and found that the total direct cost borne by the society per diabetes patient per year in the region ranged from 876 Int$ in group three countries (the poorest) to 1221 Int$ in group one countries (the wealthiest) (Kirigia *et al.*, 2009). Using country-by-country data from 193 countries, researchers estimated that the direct cost borne by the society on diabetic care in SSA in 2010 was responsible for about 7% of the total expenditure on health in the region (Zhang *et al.*, 2010). Based on secondary data and models from other countries, in 1991, researchers estimated that the total direct cost for all CVD patients in South Africa was between 1.7 million ZAR to 2.1 million ZAR (Pestana *et al.*, 1996). Based on primary data on the direct cost per diabetes patient from 464 patients and secondary data regarding the prevalence of diabetes in Tanzania, researchers found that the total direct cost for all diabetes patients in Tanzania was about four million USD, accounting for approximately 8% of the total government expenditure on health in 1989–90 (Chale *et al.*, 1992).

Among the studies mentioned above on overall OOP expenditure on CNCDs in SSA, three studies also analyzed the breakdown or the driving force of OOP expenditure on CNCDs in these settings. They found that the cost of medicine and diagnosis were the major cost for CNCDs in SSA, which is aligned with one systematic review on the financial burden due to NCDs in LMICs (Kankeu *et al.*, 2013). In one study relying on data from 147 type 1 diabetic children in Sudan, the cost of insulin was equivalent to 36% of the annual OOP expenditure for type 1 diabetes (Elrayah *et al.*, 2005). Similarly, the study from Tanzania found that the annual cost of insulin for insulin-dependent patients was 156 USD in 1989–90, which accounted for 68% of their annual direct outpatient cost. This study also listed all components of cost and their contributions to the total direct outpatient and inpatient cost for diabetic care. Transport cost was found to account for only 1–2% of the total direct outpatient cost (Chale *et al.*, 1992). Another quantitative study from Nigeria found that the greatest sources of expenditure for diabetic care were pharmacy and diagnostic costs (Odili and Okwuanasor, 2012).

1.3.2 The economic impact of OOP expenditure on CNCDs in SSA

To my knowledge, no study has been conducted to assess the economic impact of OOP expenditure on CNCDs specifically on affected households in SSA. The few existing studies on catastrophic spending and impoverishment in SSA used CNCDs as one of explanatory variables influencing the odds of catastrophic spending and impoverishment. Relying on data from 800 households from the Nouna District, Burkina Faso, researchers found that the presence of a household member with chronic diseases increased the odds of catastrophic expenditure by 3.3 to 7.8 times using different thresholds of catastrophic consequence (Su *et al.*, 2006a). Similarly, based on data from the Kenyan Health Expenditure and Utilization Survey, researchers revealed that having a member with chronic diseases increase the probability of catastrophic spending by 3.56 times (Xu *et al.*, 2006b).

1.3.3 Factors that influence OOP expenditure on CNCDs in SSA

To my knowledge, no systematic study has been conducted to specifically identify factors associated with OOP expenditure on CNCDs in SSA. Some studies on expenditure analysis in SSA included CNCDs as an explanatory variable influencing the level of OOP expenditure on healthcare, but they did not specifically describe patterns and determinants of OOP spending on CNCDs (Su *et al.*, 2006b; Xu *et al.*, 2006b; Gustafsson-Wright *et al.*, 2012), or did not clearly differentiate acute from chronic conditions in their analysis of OOP expenditure (Goudge *et al.*, 2009b; Onwujekwe *et al.*, 2010). Other studies attempted to descriptively identify a few factors influencing OOP expenditure on CNCDs, though their main focus was exclusively on estimating the overall financial burden on CNCDs in the region. One aforementioned facility-based study in Tanzania found that the absolute value of OOP expenditure for CVDs was positively associated with SES in the setting (Huffman *et al.*, 2011). In Kenya, SES was found to be negatively associated with the proportion of monthly direct cost for chronic diseases to the monthly household total expenses, suggesting that the poorest household incurred the highest financial burden due to chronic diseases (Chuma *et al.*, 2007). Similarly, based on data from 46 countries in Africa, the WHO found that the poorer the country, the higher the financial burden from CNCDs borne by households in the setting (Kirigia *et al.*, 2009). However, in Tanzania, researchers found that the proportion of OOP expenditure for CVDs to the household total expenditure did not differ across SES groups (Huffman *et al.*, 2011). In addition, two studies confirmed that treating CNCDs in private facilities brought more financial burden to households than that in public facilities (Elrayah *et al.*, 2005) or shops (Chuma *et al.*, 2007). The study from Kenya also found that the expenditure for treating chronic diseases was lower in rural areas than that in urban areas (Chuma *et al.*, 2007).

1.3.4 Knowledge gap in OOP expenditure on CNCDs in SSA

Among 18 reviewed studies on OOP expenditure on CNCDs in SSA, 11 studies relied on facility-based data from patients with a clear clinical diagnosis, four used secondary data, and the remaining three used community-based data. The 11 facility-based studies could only rely on data from individuals who self-selected to seek care at formal facilities, but could not account for the cost incurred by the individuals who did not seek any formal care. Therefore, these 11 facility-based studies could not provide a complete picture of the economic burden faced by poor rural communities in relation to CNCDs (Suhrcke et al., 2006). In addition, all these facility-based studies focused on only one CNCD. The three population-based studies either focused on chronic diseases with most of their cases being HIV/AIDS (Chuma *et al.*, 2007; Gustafsson-Wright *et al.*, 2012), or estimated the total OOP health expenditure for people both with CNCDs and without, which was not easy to obtain the accurate financial burden due to CNCDs borne by the household (Gustafsson-Wright *et al.*, 2012; Tagoe, 2013). Therefore, specific population-based study on OOP expenditure on CNCDs, especially on a broader range of CNCDs, in SSA is lacking.

Meanwhile, no systematic study is available on determinants of OOP expenditure on CNCDs in the region. A few selected studies identified very limited factors associated with OOP expenditure on CNCDs in SSA: SES, a country's economic development, whether the household is located in rural area, and whether the individual uses private facilities. Certain factor was found to have different effect on OOP expenditure for CNCDs. The limited evidence on determinants of OOP expenditure on CNCDs in SSA leaves very much still to be explained in terms of which and how individual, household, and health system factors influence OOP expenditure on these conditions in the region. More importantly, all of these studies relied on descriptive analysis, which made it impossible to control for possible con-founders (Elrayah *et al.*, 2005; Chuma *et al.*, 2007; Kirigia *et al.*, 2009; Huffman *et al.*, 2011). So, an analytical study on determinants of OOP expenditure on CNCDs in SSA is lacking.

In addition, no study has been conducted to estimate the economic impact of OOP expenditure on CNCDs specifically on affected households in SSA. Evidence on the economic impact of CNCDs specifically on affected households exists from other settings in LMICs (Bhojani *et al.*, 2012; Le *et al.*, 2012; Mukherjee and Koul, 2014). However, given remarkable disparities in overall social and political settings, the available evidence cannot provide direct policy guidance for SSA governments. So evidence on the economic impact of CNCDs on affected households within the settings of SSA is urgently needed.

1.4 Aim of the dissertation

As an explorative study, this population-based investigation aimed at filling the knowledge gap regarding treatment options and OOP expenditure on CNCDs in SSA by describing patterns of health seeking behavior and household OOP spending on CNCDs, and exploring their determinants among communities, as well as identifying the economic impact of OOP expenditure on CNCDs among affected households within the context of rural Malawi. Specifically, this study aimed to detect potential inequities in accessing care across population groups and identifying which factors place people at risk of incurring OOP expenditure and specifically higher OOP expenditure on CNCDs.

The specific objectives in this dissertation can be summarized as follows:
1) To explore patterns of and factors associated with health seeking behavior on CNCDs in rural Malawi.
2) To investigate patterns of, factors associated with, and the economic impact of OOP expenditure on CNCDs in rural Malawi.

1.5 Malawi, its health system and CNCDs in Malawi

1.5.1 The country

Malawi is a narrow and landlocked country located in southeastern Africa. It neighbors Tanzania, Mozambique and Zambia. From 1891 to 1964, the country was a British colony. At that time, it was called Nyasaland. After obtaining independence, the country was renamed as Malawi. The name Malawi originated from the old name of the people who lived there (Missions Atlas Project, 2011).

Malawi is now a multi-party republic, while before 1994 it was a single-party country. The National Assembly holds legislative power, elected every five years like the President. The capital Lilongwe is its largest city, followed by Blantyre and Mzuzu. Since 1996, Malawi has been divided into the Southern, Central, and Northern administrative regions, and is composed of 28 districts (Missions Atlas Project, 2011). Each district is subdivided into traditional authorities administered by chiefs. Under a traditional authority are villages, the lowest administrative unit in Malawi (Ministry of Health Malawi, 2011).

Malawi counts a population of 13.1 million people distributed over an area of 118,484 km². Of the total population, 49% are males and 51% are females. Out of the total population, 45%, 42%, and 13% live in the Southern, Central, and Northern regions respectively (National Statistical Office (Malawi), 2008). Of the total population, 15.8% live in urban areas, which is much lower than the average in SSA. In terms of population density, Malawi is one of the most densely inhabited countries in SSA with its population density estimated at 168 people per square kilometer in 2012 (Table 1.1) (World Bank, 2014b). Malawi's population is growing quickly, especially in recent years. The annual population increase rate has been estimated at 2.0% from 1987 to 1998, and 2.8% from 1998 to 2008. Malawi has a high dependency ratio, the ratio of the population below 15 or above 64 to the population aged between 15 and 64 (OECD, 2007), is estimated at 1.04 in 2008. Out of the total population, 46% are under 15 years of age (National Statistical Office (Malawi), 2008).

The United Nations ranks Malawi at the 170th position out of a total of 187 countries based on the Human Development Index, a measure of assessing a country's capability in meeting the needs of its population in terms of long and healthy lifetime, access to education, and a decent livelihood (United Nations Development Programme, 2013). Since 1980 Malawi has developed quickly. However, it is still one of the poorest countries in the world. In 2012, its per capita Gross National Income was 774 Int$ (adjusted by purchasing power parity in 2005), which was much lower than the average in SSA (Table 1.1) (United Nations Development Programme, 2013). Malawi's economy heavily depends on agriculture and the agriculture sector accounts for one third of the Gross Domestic Product (GDP). The main cash crops are tobacco, sugarcane, cotton, tea and so on. Out of the total population, 61.6% live under the World Bank poverty line of 1.25 USD a day (World Bank, 2014c).

Table 1.1: Demographic, social, economic, health status, and health financing indicators in Malawi and in Sub-Saharan Africa

	Malawi	Sub-Saharan Africa
Mean years of schooling (years) (2012) [a]	4.2	4.7
Gross national income per capita (2005 PPP $) (2012) [a]	774	2010
Human development index (2012) [a]	0.418	0.475
Urban population (% of total) (2012) [b]	15.8	36.8
Population density (per sq. km of land area) (2012) [b]	168.7	38.6

	Malawi	Sub-Saharan Africa
Literacy rate (population aged 15 and above) (%) [b,c]	72.1	70.4
Net enrollment rate at primary schools (%) [b,d]	96.9	76.3
Life expectancy at birth (years) (2012) [a]	54.8	54.9
Under-five mortality rate (per 1,000 live births) (2012) [b]	71	97.5
Mortality rate, infant (per 1,000 live births) (2013) [b]	46	63.9
Maternal mortality ratio (modeled estimate, per 100,000 live births) (2012) [b]	510	510
Health expenditure, total (% of GDP) (2012) [b]	9.2	6.5
Health expenditure per capita (current USD) (2012) [b]	24.5	96.3
Health expenditure, public (% of total health expenditure) (2012) [b]	76.5	43.9
Out-of-pocket health expenditure (% of private expenditure on health) (2012) [b]	53.6	73.0

Sources: a United Nations Development Programme, 2013.
b World Bank, 2014b.
c Literacy rate in Malawi in 2010, the average literacy rate in Sub-Saharan Africa in 2011.
d Net enrollment rate at primacy school in Malawi in 2009, net enrollment rate at primacy school in Sub-Saharan Africa in 2011.

Malawi has various ethnicities with Cheva, Lomwe, and Yao being the major ones, representing 32.6%, 16.6%, and 13.5% of the total population respectively (Central Intelligence Agency (USA), 2014). Out of the total population, around 69% are Christian, 26% are Muslim, and 5% believe in another religion or have no religion (Kohler *et al.*, 2014). Since the Malawian government started to provide free primary education to all children in 1994, the enrollment rate at primary school in Malawi has increased greatly. Its literacy rate was 72.1% in 2010 and enrollment rate at primary schools was 96.9% in 2009. Based on these two indicators, the education level in Malawi were higher than the average in SSA (Table 1.1) (World Bank, 2014b). English is the official language and Chichewa (or Chiwa) is the locally spoken language. Out of the total population, 62% are able to speak English (Missions Atlas Project, 2011).

1.5.2 Health status

Since 1990, the health status of the Malawian population has improved greatly. The life expectancy at birth in Malawi has increased from 47 years in 1990, to 55 years in 2012. The under-five mortality rate in Malawi has decreased from 218 per 1,000 live births in 1990, to 71 per 1,000 live births in 2012. Maternal mortality ratio has dropped from 910 per 100,000 live births in 1990, to 510 per 100,000 live births in 2012. In terms of under-five mortality rate, and infant mortality rate, the health status in Malawi is better than the average in SSA (Table 1.1) (World Bank, 2014b). In spite of the improvement of health status of the population, due to poverty, food insecurity, and insufficient health services with limited quality of care, the general health status of its population is still very poor, especially among those vulnerable subpopulations (Maseko, 2010). Inequities in health status also exist among different subpopulations, with the rich and highly educated enjoying higher health status (National Statistical Office (Malawi), 2011).

1.5.2.1 CNCDs in Malawi

As in other countries in SSA, communicable, maternal, perinatal and nutritional conditions are still the greatest health problem in Malawi. In 2008, these diseases accounted for 63% of all deaths in Malawi (Figure 1.4) (World Health Organization, 2011c). Still in recent years, CNCDs have been causing an increasing number of deaths and disabilities in the country (WHO, 2006). In 2008, CNCDs were estimated to account for 28% of all deaths and became the second single leading cause of deaths after HIV/AIDS. The leading causes of mortality due to CNCDs in 2008 were cardiovascular diseases, cancers, chronic respiratory diseases, and diabetes, representing 16%, 3%, 3% and 2% of all nationwide deaths respectively (Figure 1.4) (World Health Organization, 2011c).

Figure 1.4: Proportional mortality (% of total deaths, all ages) in 2008 in Malawi.

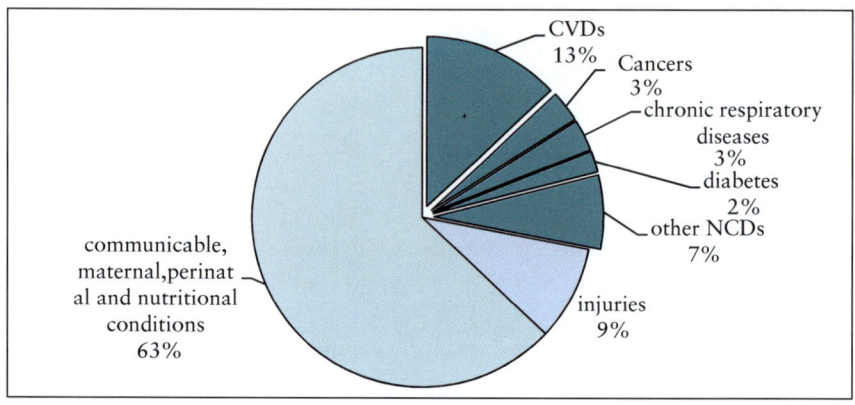

Source: World Health Organization, 2011c.

The prevalence of CNCDs and related risk factors are increasing quickly. Based on a nationwide survey on the prevalence of CNCDs and their risk factors in Malawi, 32.9%, 8.9% and 5.6% of 5206 respondents aged 25–64 suffered from high blood pressure, CVDs, and diabetes respectively. The same study found that the vast majority (93.3%) of those diagnosed with high blood pressure were unaware of their conditions. Out of 5206 respondents, 734 (14.1%) were smokers, 880 (16.9%) drank alcohol, 1141 (21.9%) were overweight, and 495 (9.5%) were not physically active (Msyamboza et al., 2011). Among 406 adults (18 years and above) randomly selected from Mwandama community in Malawi, 23% were diagnosed with hypertension by clinical measures (de Ramirez et al., 2010). Based on 18,946 new cancer cases registered between 2007 to 2010, common cancers in women were cervical cancer (accounting for 45.4% of all cases), Kaposi sarcoma (21.1%), oesophagus cancer (8.2%), breast cancer (4.6%), and non-Hodgkin lymphoma (4.1%), while common cancers in men were Kaposi sarcoma (50.7%), oesophagus cancer (16.9%), non-Hodgkin lymphoma (7.8%), prostate cancer (4.0%), and urinary bladder cancer (3.7%) (Msyamboza et al., 2012). According to the World Health Report 2004, the prevalence of asthma was estimated at 5.1% in Malawi (World Health Organization, 2004b). Another WHO study found that the mean male and female systolic blood pressure range increased from 122 mmHg and 129 mmHg to 131 mmHg and 135 mmHg, in between the years 1980 to 2008 respectively. Moreover, the mean male and female body mass index were both 21 kg/m^2 in 1980, but it increased to 22 kg/m^2 and 23 kg/m^2 respectively in 2008 (World Health Organization, 2011c).

1.5.3 The health system

1.5.3.1 Health service provision

Health service provision in Malawi depends on both public and private providers. Public providers include all facilities owned by the Ministry of Health (MoH), the Ministry of Local Government and Rural Development (MoLGRD), the Army and so on. Private sector includes private not-for-profit and for-profit facilities. The Malawian health system is mainly organized by the MoH, which is in charge of policy setting, standards and protocols development, and technical supervision. The MoH owns 63% of all health facilities in Malawi, while the Christian Health Association of Malawi (CHAM), founded in 1966 and owned by Christian-churches, owns 172 health facilities, comprising 26% of all Malawian health facilities. Over 80% of health facilities owned by CHAM are located in the rural hard to reach areas. The MoLGRD, delivering health services at district and lower level with the support under the MoH, owns another 5% of total health facilities in Malawi. The remaining 6% of Malawian health facilities are owned by others, such as the Blue Star network (a private for-profit provider) and Banja La Mtsogolo (BLM) (another private not-for-profit provider).

The health care delivery system in Malawi has three levels. The primary level of health care includes community initiatives, health posts, health centers (including dispensaries, maternities), and community hospitals (also known as rural hospitals). The primary level facilities are required to contain specific departments for ambulatory and maternal services. Community hospitals stand at a higher level than the other facilities in the primary level and are equipped to provide both primary and secondary level of care. District hospitals and CHAM facilities provide the secondary level of care. District hospitals are the referral centers for the primary level facilities and offer technical support and supervision to them. Every district is required to have one district hospital, which has 200 to 300 beds and provides in-patient and out-patient services to the local population. Central hospitals provide tertiary care, i.e. specialist referral services for district hospitals, such as obstetrics and gynecology. Currently four central hospitals exist in Malawi, which are located in Blantyre, Kamuzu (Lilongwe), Mzuzu, and Zomba. These four central hospitals do research as well as provide training and support to district hospitals. The central hospitals in Blantyre and Kamuzu are teaching hospitals because they are near to two medical colleges. The central hospital in Blantyre has the largest admission capacity of more than 1200 beds.

Officially, all health services provided through public sector are supposed to be free of charge at point of use. To further guide national policy makers and international development agencies, the MoH in 2004 defined a specific Essential Health Package (EHP) outlining a minimum package of great impact and cost-effective health interventions. The focus of the EHP is the major cause of disease burden in Malawi, especially those diseases with high incidence and prevalence among vulnerable populations. The EHP is provided free of charge at all public health facilities and at selected CHAM and BLM contracted by the MoH through Service Level Agreements (SLAs). SLAs are supposed to cover all services within the EHP, to date only maternal and child services are included in SLAs (Maseko, 2010). Till 2011, a total of 75 out of 172 CHAM facilities had signed the SLAs (Chirwa et al., 2013).

Initially, the EHP covered only the costs related to prevention and treatment of communicable, maternal, perinatal, and nutritional conditions. In 2010, the EHP was expanded to include coverage for common CNCDs, such as the screening, prevention, and treatment of cardiovascular, diabetic, and cancerous diseases, therapeutic approaches targeting forms of chronic mental illness, and the general promotion of healthy lifestyles in relation to CNCDs, as well as neglected tropical diseases (Table 1.2) (Ministry of Health Malawi, 2011).

Table 1.2: Conditions covered by the current EHP

	Conditions covered by the EHP
Initial designed EHP in 2004	HIV/AIDS
	Acute respiratory infections (ARI)
	Malaria
	Diarrheal diseases
	Perinatal conditions
	Tuberculosis
	Malnutrition
	Vaccine preventable diseases
	Eye, ear and skin infections
Later inclusions in 2010	Common CNCDs (e.g. CVDs, diabetes, and cancers)
	Neglected Tropical Diseases

Source: Ministry of Health, 2011.
Notes: EHP = Essential Health Package; CVDs = cardiovascular diseases.

1.5.3.2 Health financing

The country's health financing structure relies on general tax revenue and external donor funds. External resources for health accounts for 53.6% of total expenditure on health in Malawi (World Health Organization, 2014b). The health expenditure per capita in Malawi stands at 24.5 USD, equivalent to 9.2% of the GDP (World Bank, 2014b). This country spends a higher proportion of its GDP on health, though its absolute per capita health expenditure is lower than the average in SSA. Public health expenditure in Malawi accounts for 76.5% of total health expenditure, which is much higher than the average in SSA. OOP health expenditure in Malawi takes up 53.6% of private health expenditure, which is much lower than the average in SSA (Table 1.1) (World Bank, 2014b). In this state-funded health system where health care is supposed to be free of charge at all public facilities and at selected not-for-profit facilities through SLAs, no nation-wide complementary health insurance exists. Only several companies have private medical aids that can cover their employees' health care costs. The major provider of such medical aid is the Medical Aid Society of Malawi (Maseko, 2010; Abiiro et al., 2014).

1.5.3.3 Challenges of the health system

The Malawian health system has long been facing some persistent challenges: inadequate financing, lack of drugs and other medical supplies, insufficient human resources, limited quality of services, inequity in accessing care and so on (Ministry of Health Malawi, 2011). In recent years, the emerging CNCDs together with still highly prevalent acute communicable diseases bring new challenges to the Malawian health system. These problems in the health system are not well solved even after the implementation of the EHP in 2004, which affect the role of the EHP in improving the performance of Malawian health system (Bowie and Mwase, 2011; Chirwa et al., 2013). The Malawi Demographic and Health Survey revealed that from 2004 to 2010 infant, child, and maternal mortality dropped only modestly (National Statistical Office (Malawi), 2005, 2011).

Underfunding and the extensive shortage of drugs and staff are the main constraints to the successful implementation of the EHP, which cause the vast majority of services required by the EHP to be underprovided or not existent in reality (Bowie et al., 1995; Mueller et al., 2011). One recent quantitative study from Malawi found that one of the most basic and vital drugs for bacterial infections, Cotrimoxazole, were only available in 27% of public facilities surveyed (Mueller et al., 2011). In terms of human resources, Malawi has the worst situation in SSA (Maseko, 2010) with every 100,000 Malawian population having 1.5 general and specialist medical practitioners and 27 nurses (Africa Health Workforce Observatory, 2009). Only nearly half of expected man days of these insufficient health staff are available. Trainings are their main reason for absence. In spite of the trainings, the ability of health staff to diagnose and treat common and vital diseases remains limited (Mueller et al., 2011). In addition, public facilities in Malawi are considered to have poor quality of care. If people can afford the cost of private facilities, they prefer private facilities to public facilities

(Abiiro *et al.*, 2014). Despite being an officially free health system, inequity in access still exists in Malawi with the vulnerable population ending up using less care (Muula and Maseko, 2006; Chibwana *et al.*, 2009; Mueller *et al.*, 2011; Makaula *et al.*, 2012).

2. Methods

2.1 Study setting

2.1.1 The demographic, economic, and cultural context in the study area

I conducted my study in Thyolo, Chiradzulu, and Mulanje, three rural districts in Southern Malawi (Figure 2.1). These three districts cover an area of 4,538 square meters, accounting for 4.8% of the country area. Approximately 1.4 million people live in these three districts, equivalent to 11% of the country population. Populations live relatively intensively in these three districts, compared with the national average population density (Table 2.1) (National Statistical Office Malawi 2008).

Figure 2.1: The map of Thyolo, Chiradzulu, and Mulanje districts.

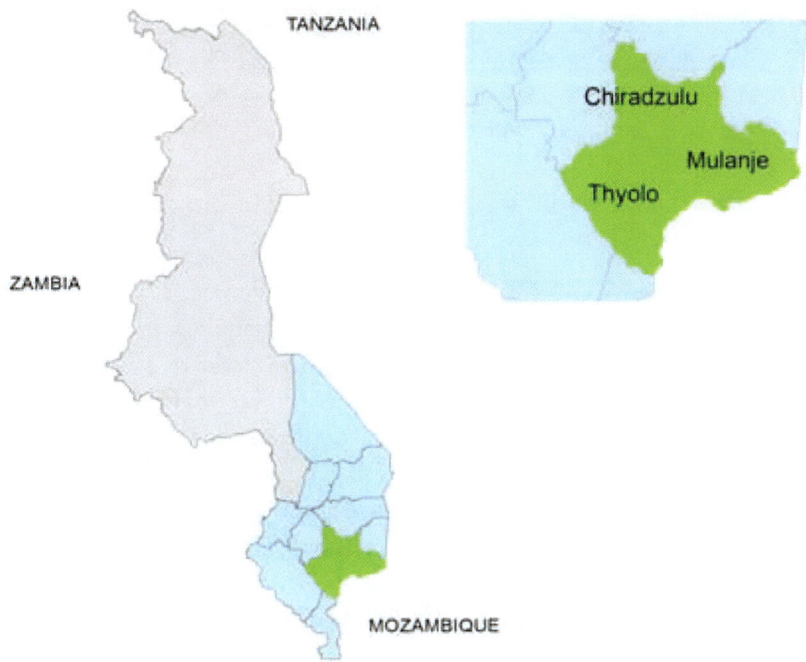

All these three districts are basically rural areas with a few semi-urban settlements. Their economy is based on agriculture. In these three districts, people rely on subsistence farming. In Mulanje and Thyolo, tea is their major economic crop and a vast majority of people work in tea farms. Since people in these districts live on farming, which is prone to drought and flooding and thus represents an instable source of income, the poverty incidence is much higher there than the national average level. However, the Gini index, a measure of inequality in income distribution among the population with 0 representing completely equality and 1 representing completely inequality (World Bank, 2015), is much smaller in these three districts than that in the whole area of Malawi. This means that income is more equally distributed in these districts than that of the whole area of Malawi, though the population in these areas is poorer (Table 2.1) (National Statistical Office (Malawi), 2012a). In addition, similar to the whole country, household food consumption accounts for more than 55% of total household consumption in these three districts and more than 45% of the population there are facing food shortage. The literacy rate in Thyolo, Chirazulu, and Mulanje is 66.7%, 76.4%, and 62.3% respectively (Table 2.1) (National Statistical Office (Malawi), 2012a). People in these three districts share the same culture, which is based on matriarchy. The major ethnic group in these three districts is Alomwe.

2.1.2 Health status and health service provision in the study area

Compared with the national level, child mortality rate, infant mortality rate, and under-five mortality rate are all higher in these three districts while life expectancy at birth for both male and female is lower. All these indicators show that people in these three districts have a worse health condition than an average Malawian (Table 2.1) (National Statistical Office (Malawi), 2012b). In addition, studies have shown that the proportion of chronically ill (including HIV, tuberculosis, chronic malaria, and CNCDs) in Chiradzulu was more than twice as large as the national average (Table 2.1) (National Statistical Office (Malawi), 2012b).

In line with national health financing structure and policies, the EHP with the expanded coverage of the most common CNCDs is provided free of charge at all public facilities and at selected CHAM and BLM in these three areas. At the time of the study, these three districts counted a total of 60 public health facilities, 16 private not-for-profit health facilities operated by CHAM, and six private for profit health facilities. All these facilities provide primary or secondary level of health care. No central hospital providing tertiary health care exists in these three districts. More than 95% of the population live within an 8 km radius of health facilities in these three districts with all of them outnumbering the national average level by more than 10% (Table 2.1) (Ministry of Health Malawi, 2011).

Table 2.1: Demographic, social, economic, and health status indicators in Thyolo, Chiradzulu, and Mulanje districts

	Malawi	Thyolo	Chiradzulu	Mulanje
Population (2008) [a]	13,066,320	587,455	290,946	525,429
Female / male (2008) [a]	51/49	52/48	53/47	53/47
Land area (sq.km.) [a]	94,276	1,715	767	2,056
Population density (per sq. km of land area) (2008) [a]	139	343	379	256
Poverty incidence (%) (2011) [b]	52.4	64.9	63.5	68.6
Gini index (2011) [b]	0.452	0.317	0.377	0.384
Consumption per person per year (MWK) (2011) [b]	54,568	52,274	57,750	38,211
Consumption per capita per year on food to consumption per capita per year (%) (2011) [b]	56.3	64.4	55.6	58.6
Proportion of the population that faced food shortage in the past 12 months (%) (2011) [b]	49.1	57.7	45.0	52.9
Literacy rate (population aged 15 and above) (%) (2011) [b]	65.4	66.7	76.4	62.3
Average household size (2008) [a]	4.4	4.1	4.1	4.1
Proportion of the population living within 8 km radius of a health facility (%) (2011) [c]	81	95	98	96
Health status indicators				
Child mortality rate (per 1,000 live births) (2008) [d]	59		69	78

	Malawi	Thyolo	Chiradzulu	Mulanje
Infant mortality rate (per 1,000 live births) (2008) [d]	87		98	107
Under-five mortality rate (per 1,000 live births) (2008) [d]	140		159	176
Life expectancy at birth for male (year) (2008) [d]	48.3		44.1	41
Life expectancy at birth for female (year) (2008) [d]	51.4		46.9	45
Proportion of chronically ill (%) (2008) [d]	5.0		11.4	4.1

Sources: [a] National Statistical Office (Malawi), 2008.
[b] National Statistics Office (Malawi), 2012a.
[c] Ministry of Health (Malawi), 2011.
[d] National Statistics Office (Malawi), 2012b.

2.2 Data and data collection

2.2.1 Sampling

I used data from the first round of a panel household health survey on a total sample of 1199 households, spread across 77 villages. The sample included both households where one of the adults was a member of the local Bvumbwe Savings and Credit Cooperative (SACCO) (n = 691) and households where no adult was a member of the same SACCO (n = 525). The household was defined as all the people usually living together in a house and sharing meals, expenses and living arrangements (excluding paid servants for the household or short-term visitors (less than six months)) (World Bank, 2012; National Statistical Office (Malawi), 2011).

Sampling decisions were informed by the long term need of the panel household health survey to evaluate the impact of a future health insurance product channeled through the Bvumbwe SACCO, the only SACCO present in the study area and affiliated with the national Malawian Union of Saving and Credit Cooperatives.

Sampling relied on a two-stage procedure: first, all households where at least one adult was a member of the Byumbwe SACCO was interviewed in the study area. Non-SACCO households were selected using a random-route method. Selection was based on proximity to the treatment households and using them as the starting points: For every second treatment household, the interviewers needed to interview one control household. They chose a random direction decided by spinning a bottle outside the compound of the treatment household and then went to interview either the first or the third house (in a sequence of 1st, 3rd, 1st,...) of the treatment household. However, the distinction between SACCO and non-SACCO households is irrelevant for this study since I used data from the baseline survey round, before any intervention had taken place.

2.2.2 The questionnaire

2.2.2.1 The questionnaire for the panel survey

The panel survey questionnaire comprised both household and individual questions. Household questions included household socio-demographic and economic background. Individual questions included: health status; reported illness patterns (for acute, chronic, and maternal conditions); health seeking behavior, related spending, and sources of expenditure; membership and use of financial product; membership and trust in local institutions; businesses, investments and investment risks; questions on utilization of digital devices for data collection; and solidarity attitudes.

Each member of the household was interviewed individually for individual questions. Household head was responsible to answer household questions. Mothers or the closest caretaker responded as proxy for children below the age of 14. For children between 14 and 17, their parents can decide whether children in the age range can answer individual questions.

The questionnaire of the panel survey was first developed in English by the team at the University of Heidelberg. Then research associates at the Research for Equity and Community Health Trust (REACH Trust) translated the questionnaire from English into Chichewa. Then the Chichewa version of the questionnaire was retranslated into English by other associates from the same organization. Last, I, together with other colleagues from the University of Heidelberg, compared the original English version and the re-translation version of the questionnaire and found the inconsistency between these two versions, which was corrected by the team before field work started.

2.2.2.2 The questionnaire for CNCDs

To ensure the completeness of reported information on CNCDs, the section of the questionnaire for CNCDs was designed to collect illness information based on both medical definitions (diseases or disorders related to clinical symptoms) and illness experience (impairment or disabilities) according to WHO's International Classification (World Health Organization, 1980) (Appendix 8.2). In line with previous studies on chronic diseases (Gans, 1988; Su et al., 2006a; Chuma et al., 2007), the questionnaire on CNCDs started with one question: whether the respondent was experiencing any illness or symptom that lasted longer than three months or any illness or complaint that occurred earlier in a respondent's life and continued to affect the individual's health status at the time of the interview. Interviewers were trained to identify reported illnesses or complaints based on their description by the respondents and coded them either as primary and secondary diagnoses or symptoms. The reported information on chronic diagnoses and symptoms was further categorized into one of 10 non-communicable illness categories, based on the WHO categories commonly used for reporting the global disease burden of non-communicable diseases (World Health Organization, 2008a). The simplified grouping algorithm allowed interviewers to assign listed non-communicable disorders and symptoms into the 10 CNCD categories (Appendix 8.1), which the interviewer was required to carry at each interview. The algorithm was reviewed and adjusted by clinical experts prior to data collection under the assumption that information on illness-related data was complete.

Once respondents reported one or more chronic illness or complaint (i.e. lead and secondary complaints), the interviewers continued to ask a series of additional questions on utilization of health care services and OOP expenditure related to these chronic conditions. In line with prior research (Su et al., 2006b; Abegunde and Stanciole, 2008; Goudge et al., 2009b; Onwujekwe et al., 2010; Rahman et al., 2013), information on health service utilization and OOP expenditure was limited to a four-week recall period (Appendix 8.2).

2.2.3 Field procedures

2.2.3.1 Interviewer training and pre-testing

Prior to field work, the interviewers received an eight-day consecutive training done by the team at the University of Heidelberg. Besides the introduction of all sections in the questionnaire, the training also taught the interviewers how to apply digital devices for data collection. During the process of training, the interviewers brought up some suggestions on the questionnaire in both the English and the Chichewa versions, which helped the questionnaire improve.

At the end of the training, the questionnaire was pre-tested in the rural area of Lilongwe, which is a different area from the study setting so that the households attending the pre-test were different from the subsequent panel sample. The core team from the University of Heidelberg accompanied the interviewers in the pre-test in order to identify problems and to provide guidance when needed. The questionnaire was improved during the pre-test.

2.2.3.2 Field organization

The field work team consisted of nine interviewers, three supervisors, and one field coordinator. The interviewers were organized in teams with each team including three interviewers and one supervisor. Supervisors were selected for their extensive experience in data collection in the field of public health. Besides interviewing the respondents, supervisors needed to contact the households and reserve the time of interview, prepare digitalized data collection for other interviewers, check the completeness and accuracy of the completed questionnaires done by the interviewers, and send the checked data to the server as well as to the coordinator.

2.2.4 Data collection

Data collection lasted from August 27th to October 20th, 2012. A fully digitalized system was used for data collection by means of tablet computers and direct data transfer over mobile phone networks, which ensured high quality data through complex built-in filters and logic checks.

Before interviewing respondents, interviewers explained the aim of the survey and asked for consent from the respondents (Appendix 8.3). The interview would only continue when the respondent agreed and signed the consent form in Chichewa. This study obtained ethical approval from the Ethikkommission der Medizinischen Fakultät Heidelberg (the Ethical Committee of the Faculty of Medicine, Heidelberg University, Germany) and the National Health Sciences Research Committee, Ministry of Health, Malawi.

2.3 Variables and their measurement

Table 2.2 presents a list of all outcome and explanatory variables included in the analysis of health seeking behavior and OOP expenditure and their measurement. Both the outcome variables for the analysis of health seeking behavior and OOP expenditure were defined at the individual level. All expenditure information, whether related to the outcome or to the explanatory variables, is expressed in the local currency, Malawian Kwacha (MWK) with MWK 280 being equivalent to about 1 US Dollar at time of data collection. To facilitate data analysis, especially in the empirical model of both health seeking behavior and OOP expenditure, I divided all monetary amounts related to explanatory variables by 1,000 using '1,000 MWK' as the adjusted unit (Acock, 2008).

2.3.1 The outcome variables

The outcome variable in the analysis of health seeking behavior was defined as the health seeking option among those reporting at least one CNCD, and included three categories: no care, informal care (traditional care and home treatment), and formal care (care provided by public facilities, CHAM and private for-profit facilities). The distinction in three categories (no care, informal care, and formal care) was deemed to be essential, given the limited knowledge available on health seeking related to CNCDs in SSA and the subsequent exploratory nature of this study. From a conceptual point of view, this decision was justified by the desire to reflect as accurately as possible the actual choice set facing local communities.

The outcome variable in the analysis of OOP expenditure was defined as the four-week individual OOP expenditure incurred in the process of seeking care, including medical and travel expenditure. OOP medical expenditure included consultation fees, laboratory tests, and drugs, whether they had been incurred for routine care or for an acute illness episode related to an underlying CNCD. Travel expenditure included only direct transportation costs, but excluded the opportunity cost associated with seeking care.

In addition, derived from the variable of OOP expenditure, I looked at catastrophic spending and impoverishment due to OOP expenditure on CNCDs. Catastrophic spending due to CNCDs was defined as the share of household out-of-pocket health expenditure caused by CNCDs in relation to household non-subsistence expenditure (total household expenditure minus expenditure for basic subsistence needs) once exceeding a given threshold level (Xu *et al.*, 2003). In practice, in line with previous studies (Xu *et al.*, 2003; Su *et al.*, 2006a; Chuma and Maina, 2012; Kwesiga *et al.*, 2015), I used food expenditure as a proxy of a household's basic subsistence needs. Also in line with prior research (Chuma and Maina, 2012), I set the threshold levels in this study at 10%, 25%, and 40%. Meanwhile, impoverishment due to CNCDs was defined as the difference in poverty rate before paying for CNCD care (i.e. pre-payment poverty rate) and after making such payments (i.e. post-payment poverty rate), i.e. the percentage of non-poor households falling into poverty due to direct costs associated with CNCDs (O'Donnell *et al.*, 2007; Jiang *et al.*, 2012). Due to the fact that information on the national poverty line for 2012 was not available in Malawi, I used the international poverty line, $1.25 per person per day (Ravallion *et al.*, 2008). I converted the $1.25 per person per day into the local currency using the official 2012 purchasing power parity exchange rate of 88.17 (World Bank, 2015). This yielded a poverty line of 3306.4 MWK per person per month.

To counter the effect of extreme cases of expenditure data, the descriptive analysis of OOP expenditure relied on trimmed means. By excluding the smallest 5% and largest 5% of all cases in a sample, this approach allows for a better measurement of central tendency (Osborn, 2000).

Table 2.2: Variables, their measurements, and expected sign of explanatory variables

Variable	Measurement	Expected signs in the HSB model		Expected sign in the OOP expenditure model	
		Formal care vs. No-care	Informal care vs. No-care	Probability of positive expenditure	Determinants of level of expenditure
Health seeking options	0=no care 1=informal care 2=formal care	N/A	N/A	N/A	N/A
Individual four-week OOP expenditure (including medical and transportation cost) (MWK)	Continuous variable	N/A	N/A	N/A	N/A
Age (years)	Continuous variable	+/-	+/-	+/-	+/-
Being household head	0 = No 1 = Yes	+	+	+	+
Sex	0 = Male 1 = Female	+/-	+/-	+/-	+/-
Ethnicity	0 = Other 1 = Alomwe	+	+	+	+
Perceiving CNCD as serious	0 = No 1 = Yes	+	+	+	+
Duration of CNCDs (years)	Continuous variable	+/-	+/-	+/-	+/-
CNCDs targeted by screening program	0 = No 1 = Yes	+	-	-	-
Six-month per capita household expenditure (MWK 1000)	Continuous variable, used in the analysis for health seeking behavior	+	+	N/A	N/A

Variable	Measurement	Expected signs in the HSB model		Expected sign in the OOP expenditure model	
		Formal care vs. No-care	Informal care vs. No-care	Probability of positive expenditure	Determinants of level of expenditure
Four-week per capita household expenditure (MWK 1000)	Used as continuous variable in two part model for OOP expenditure; Categorized into quartiles (1= lowest SES; 4= highest SES) for descriptive analysis for OOP expenditure	N/A	N/A	+	+
Household head literacy	0 = No 1 = Yes	+	+	+	+
Proportion of people with CNCDs within the household	Used as dichotomous variable in the analysis for health seeking behavior (0 = Household with less than 50% household members reporting a CNCD; 1 = Household with 50% or more household members reporting a CNCD); used as continuous variable in the analysis for OOP expenditure	-	-	-	-
Distance to nearest health facility (km)	Continuous variable	+/-	+/-	+/-	+/-
Use of formal care	0 = No 1 = Yes	N/A	N/A	-	-

Notes: HSB = health seeking behavior; OOP = out-of-pocket; N/A = not applicable.

2.3.2 The explanatory variables

I included individual, household, and health system characteristics as explanatory variables in the analysis of health seeking behavior and OOP expenditure. Individual level characteristics included age, sex, ethnicity, being household head or not, duration of illness (in years), perceived severity (measured as the inability to conduct daily activities), whether respondents were suffering from a CNCD targeted by screening programs available through the EHP. I categorized ethnicity according to whether people belonged to the major ethnic group (Alomwe) in the study area. Since CNCDs include a rather inhomogeneous range of diseases, which due to small numbers could not be entered as such in the model, I computed a variable which re-assigned the 10 CNCD categories used to recall illness into one of two chronic disease classes: CNCDs targeted by screening programs available through the EHP and CNCDs not targeted by screening programs or targeted by case management programs only (Table 2.3). The re-classification distinguished two major groups of CNCDs: (i) CNCDs with early detectable subclinical components where the individual is unaware of any illness symptoms although a clear underlying pathology is present and clinical signs of subclinical illness identifiable by means of early clinical diagnostic measures (available within the Malawian EHP, such as blood pressure checks for hypertension screening), and modifiable by early risk factor modulation; (ii) CNCDs without significant subclinical component that is identifiable by early diagnostic measures and thus only amenable by late diagnostic or therapeutic measures once the individual is aware of symptoms and/or complaints due to overt clinical manifestation. The first group is hereafter referred to as "early detectable CNCDs", the latter group as "established CNCDs". The few respondents (n=17) who reported both types of CNCDs were categorized into the established CNCD group, assuming this alternative would dominate health seeking choices as I consider an individual's awareness of illness symptoms to constitute a stronger incentive to seeking health care compared to an individual's awareness of subclinical signs in the absence of actual symptoms. The rationale behind this classification in the analysis of health seeking behavior is that treatment behavior is likely to be shaped by a person's awareness and motivation either to limit disease progression even in the absence of physical symptoms (to be expected in case of early detectable CNCDs), or to alleviate symptoms after overt disease manifestation (to be expected in case of established CNCDs). While the rationale for such division in the analysis of OOP expenditure rested on the hypothesis that expenditure incurred may differ across the two sets of conditions, given that the former set can be targeted ahead of symptomatic manifestations while the latter cannot.

Table 2.3: CNCDs re-classification

Established CNCDs	Early detectable CNCDs
Chronic musculoskeletal conditions & chronic pain syndromes	Chronic cardiovascular conditions
Chronic respiratory conditions	Malignant neoplastic conditions
Chronic sense organ conditions	Chronic endocrine conditions
Chronic neuropsychiatric conditions	
Chronic digestive conditions	
Chronic skin or oral conditions	
Chronic genitourinary conditions	
Other chronic problems	

Household level factors included SES, household head literacy, and proportion of people with CNCDs living in the household. In line with prior research (Gnawali *et al.*, 2009; Pokhrel *et al.*, 2010), I used six-month per capita household expenditure data as a proxy of household SES in the analysis of health seeking behavior. In line with other studies (Chuma *et al.*, 2007; Goudge *et al.*, 2009b; Rahman *et al.*, 2013; Yardim *et al.*, 2014) and in order to align with the analysis of the OOP expenditure intensity ratio, the four-week per capita household expenditure was used as a proxy of household SES in the analysis of OOP expenditure. The survey collected expenditure data on various items (e.g. food, alcohol, clothing, housing, transportation, communication, entertainment, education, personal care, insurance, transfers and remittances) at the collective household level. To take into account underlying differences due to household size, per capita expenditure was computed by dividing aggregated household expenditure by the number of household members. To ensure independence from the outcome variables in the analysis of health seeking behavior and OOP expenditure, my measurement of expenditure did not include healthcare expenditure. Proportion of people with CNCDs within the household was coded as a dummy variable according to whether a household having 50% or more household members reporting a CNCD in the analysis of health seeking behavior, while in the analysis of OOP expenditure proportion of people with CNCDs within the household was set as a continuous variable.

Health system characteristics included distance to nearest facility in both the analysis of health seeking behavior and OOP expenditure. In the analysis of OOP expenditure, health system factors also included use of formal care. Global Position System coordinates were collected for every household and for all formal health care facilities in the area. Distance to nearest facility was approximated by straight line distances between household and formal health care facilities. As mentioned before, an individual was defined as having used formal care if he/she had sought care at a public facility, at a non-for-profit facility, or at a private facility.

2.4 Analytical frameworks to model health seeking behavior and healthcare expenditure

2.4.1 Analytical options for modelling health seeking behavior

The modelling of health seeking behavior is done according to choice models (e.g. whether to seek care or which specific care was chosen) (Lawson, 2004). Choice set in choice models must be mutually exclusive, exhaustive, and finite. Choice models include two types of data: revealed preference data and stated preference data. Health seeking behavior data belong to the former (Hensher $et\ al.$, 2005; Train, 2009).

For a rational individual i, when facing j alternatives, he/she chooses the alternative that brings him/her the greatest utility. The utility U_{ij} can be expressed as the sum of an observable deterministic component, V_{ij}, and an unobserved random component ε_{ij}:

$$U_{ij} = V_{ij} + \varepsilon_{ij}$$

where V_{ij} is a function of the attributes of the individual, z_i, also called case-specific regressors, and the attributes of the alternatives, x_{ij}, also called alternative-specific regressors (Ryan $et\ al.$, 2001; Cameron and Trivedi, 2010):

$$V_{ij} = x'_{ij}\beta + z'_i\gamma_j$$

The possibility that individual i chooses alternative j can be expressed as follows:

$$P_{ij} = P\left(U_{ij} > U_{ik}\right) = P\left(V_{ij} + \varepsilon_{ij} > V_{ik} + \varepsilon_{ik}\right) = P\left(\varepsilon_{ik} - \varepsilon_{ij} < V_{ij} - V_{ik}\right) \forall j \neq k$$

Table 2.4: Common discrete choice models

		The distribution of random terms	The assumption of IIA	Wide- or long-form data	Stata command
Binomial choice models	Logit	Logistically distributed	–	Wide- form	logit
	Probit	Normally distributed	–	Wide- form	probit
Multinomial choice models	Multinomial logit model	iid with the type I extreme-value distribution	The assumption of IIA holds.	Wide-form	mlogit
	Conditional logit model	iid with the type I extreme-value distribution	The assumption of IIA holds.	Long-form	clogit, asclogit
	Nested logit model	A generalization of the type I extreme-value distribution	Relax the assumption of IIA partially.	Long-form	nlogit
	Mixed logit model	With type II extreme-value distribution	Relax the assumption of IIA fully.	Long-form	mixlogit

Sources: Baum, 2006; Cameron and Trivedi, 2005, 2010; Christiadi and Cushing, 2007; Hensher et al., 2005.

In the following, I list several common choice models (Table 2.4). How to choose an appropriate choice model depends on the nature of the data structure (binary or multinomial outcomes as well as wide- or long-form data structure, i.e. whether to include alternative-specific regressors) and the distribution of the random terms $\varepsilon_{ik} - \varepsilon_{ij}$ (Cameron and Trivedi, 2005, 2010).

2.4.1.1 Binomial choice models

The logit model is a common binary choice model. It assumes that $\varepsilon_{ik} - \varepsilon_{ij}$ are logistically distributed (Table 2.4). Under the logit model, for individual i, the probability of taking alternative j can be expressed as follows (Cameron and Trivedi, 2005; Baum, 2006):

$$P_{ij} = \frac{1}{1 + exp\left[-(V_{ij} - V_{ik})\right]}$$

The probit model is another common binary choice model. It assumes that $\varepsilon_{ik} - \varepsilon_{ij}$ is normally distributed (Table 2.4). Under the probit model, for individual i, the probability of taking alternative j can be expressed as follows (Baum, 2006):

$$P_{ij} = \Phi(V_{ij} - V_{ik})$$

The coefficients derived from the logit model are much easier and more straightforward to interpret than those of the probit model as the coefficients of the logit model represent log odds ratios (Cameron and Trivedi, 2010).

2.4.1.2 Multinomial choice models

The multinomial logit model (MNL) is one of the most widely used multinomial choice models thanks to its simple computation and easily interpretable coefficients. MNL requires $\varepsilon_{ik} - \varepsilon_{ij}$ to be independently and identically distributed (iid) with the type I extreme-value distribution. MNL needs the assumption of independence of irrelevant alternatives (IIA) to hold. IIA means that the correlation between each pair of the random terms within the model is equal to zero, i.e. the odds ratio between any pair of choices is independent of adding or omitting any other choice. The stata command of MNL is 'mlogit' (Cameron and Trivedi, 2005). Estimates obtained through MNL can cause a higher joint probability for choices that have similarity (Maddala, 1983). In addition, MNL is based on wide-form data, i.e. it can only have case-specific regressors, z_i, since when using MNL alternative characteristics are only available for the alternative that the decision maker has chosen, but not for the other alternatives (Table 2.4). Under MNL, for individual i, the probability of taking alternative j can be expressed as follows (Cameron and Trivedi, 2010):

$$P_{ij} = \frac{\exp(z_i'\gamma_j)}{\sum_{j=1}^{J}\exp(z_i'\gamma_j)}$$

The conditional logit model (CL) is another common multinomial logit model. CL can have both case-specific regressors, z_i, and alternative-specific regressors, x_{ij}. CL is based on long-form data. Similar to MNL, CL also requires $\varepsilon_{ik} - \varepsilon_{ij}$ to be iid with the type I extreme-value distribution. The assumption of IIA needs to hold in CL (Christiadi and Cushing, 2007). The stata command of CL is 'clogit' or 'asclogit'. Case-specific variables cannot be directly used as explanatory variables when using the command of 'clogit'. Instead, case-specific variables can be set as interactions with alternative-specific variables using the command of 'clogit' (Table 2.4). Under CL, for individual i, the probability of taking alternative j can be expressed as follows (Cameron and Trivedi, 2010):

$$P_{ij} = \frac{\exp(x_{ij}'\beta + z_i'\gamma_j)}{\sum_{j=1}^{J}\exp(x_{ij}'\beta + z_i'\gamma_j)}$$

The nested logit model (NL) is less restrictive than MNL and CL. It assumes the random terms to be with a generalization of the type I extreme-value distribution. The data structure in NL needs to be hieratical. NL only relaxes the assumption of IIA within groups (i.e. the random terms in NL are correlated within group), but not across groups (i.e. the random terms in NL are uncorrelated across groups). MNL is nested within NL. If the random terms within groups are independent, NL reduces to MNL (Dor et al., 1987; Yip et al., 1998; Brown and Theoharides, 2009). CL is also a special case of NL where both the random terms within groups and across groups are independent. NL is based on long-form data (Hensher et al., 2005; Christiadi and Cushing, 2007). The stata command of NL is 'nlogit' (Table 2.4) (Cameron and Trivedi, 2010).

The mixed logit model relaxes the assumption of IIA by allowing the coefficients in the model to vary across different choice makers. The random terms in mixed logit model are with type II extreme-value distribution.

Allowing the coefficients in the model to differ implies that people may have heterogeneous preferences (Hensher *et al.*, 2005). The stata command of mixed logit model is 'mixlogit'. Similar to the command of 'clogit', the command of 'mixlogit' does not directly include case-specific regressors as explanatory variables. Instead, it allows case-specific variables to interact with alternative-specific variables (Table 2.4) (Cameron and Trivedi, 2010).

2.4.2 The model that I chose to analyze health seeking behavior in this study

Considering that the outcome variable in the analysis of health seeking behavior included three answer categories, this study could not use binomial choice models with simple dichotomous alternative formal care vs. all else (Bourne 2010; Pokhrel et al. 2010), but relied on multinomial choice models. Taking into account that MNL is one of the most frequently used model in studies on health seeking behavior (Bolduc *et al.*, 1996; Borah, 2006), the choice set (no care, formal care, informal care) in my study had little similarity, and my data did not contain alternative-specific regressors, this study gave priority to MNL to model treatment options on CNCDs.

To apply MINL, IIA must hold (Cameron and Trivedi, 2010). I checked the assumption of IIA for MNL using both the Hausman test and the Small-Hsiao test (Hidayat *et al.*, 2004; Dong *et al.*, 2008). Both the Hausman and the Small-Hsiao test confirmed that the model did not violate the IIA assumption (all $p>0.05$). This indicated that MNL was allowed to use to model health seeking behavior in this study. The fact that my study used MNL to model health seeking options for CNCDs was in line with a few previous studies on treatment options in SSA (Hjortsberg, 2003; Su *et al.*, 2006b; Dong *et al.*, 2008).

2.4.3 Analytical options for modelling healthcare expenditure

Understanding patterns and determinants of healthcare expenditure is of importance to understanding the distribution of financial burden of diseases among populations and thus of help to draft policy recommendations to local policy makers. Talking about expenditure implies two levels of discussion: expenditure within a fixed period of time (e.g. expenditure of strokes within the last month or year) and expenditure per episode or per lifetime of a certain disease (e.g. lifetime cost of ischemic stroke). The latter belongs to survival data, i.e. right-censored data, which is totally different from the former in nature, and needs survival analysis methods to be analyzed (Lang *et al.*, 2009). Considering my expenditure data belonged to the former case, expenditure data collected with a four-week recall period, the analytical options that I summarize below are all only adequate to model expenditure within a fixed period of time.

The difficulty of analyzing healthcare expenditure data lies with their distribution: they are typically right-skewed and usually contain a mass of observations at zero expenditure. Generally, two different approaches are commonly used to model determinants of healthcare expenditure: single-equation modeling and multi-part modeling (including two-part model) (Basu and Manning, 2009; Hill and Miller, 2010). The majority of the single-equation models and all of the multi-part models that I introduce below have been developed to deal with the analytical difficulties caused by the distribution of healthcare expenditure data. Single-equation models include ordinary least square (OLS), Box-Cox transformation, generalized linear model (GLM), and extended estimating equations (EEE). As to multi-part models, I first review the two-part model, followed by an extension of the two-part model and a generalized version of multipart model. Currently, no single method is dominantly the best choice for all cases of healthcare expenditure analysis. The proper method to analyze expenditure need to consider the nature and distribution of the specific expenditure data available (Basu and Manning, 2009). For each model listed below, I summarize the strengths, limitations and application conditions.

2.4.3.1 Single-equation modelling

2.4.3.1.1 OLS

OLS model, a traditional single-equation and a basic linear regression model, remains a popular alternative to many pragmatic researchers. It is defined as the method which minimizes the total of squared vertical distances from the observed outcome (y) in the dataset to the predicted value of outcome ($\hat{y}$) by the regression estimation. The formula of the OLS is listed below:

$$E(y|x) = \alpha + \beta_i x_i$$

The OLS has its own values: it is easy for application and has no transformation problem since it uses the raw-scale value of healthcare expenditure data. But it overemphasizes influential outliers when healthcare expenditure data are skewed and have a heavy right tail, which is the common case for healthcare expenditure data. To explain it in detail, the β_i hat estimated through the OLS can be expressed as below:

$$\hat{\beta}_1 = \beta_i + (X'X)^{-1}X'\varepsilon$$

when some $|\varepsilon|$'s and X's are extremely large and dominant, the β_i hat deviates greatly away from β_i.

In addition, the β_i hat obtained through the OLS are not robust in a small or medium dataset given skewness and kurtosis of the underlying data distribution, as well as relatively inefficient given the heteroscedasticity (Fu *et al.*, 2011).

To address the issues of skewness and heteroscedasticity, i.e. the issues that the OLS cannot solve, two additional types of single-equation models were developed: one based on the transformation of the outcome variable, i.e. Box-Cox transformation (with logarithmic transformation being the most common case), the other one based on the GLM (Manning and Mullahy, 2001).

2.4.3.1.2 Box-Cox transformation

The Box-Cox transformation is widely applied, especially the log(y) version, in data analysis. I list the formula of Box-Cox transformation as following (Box and Cox, 1964):

$$y^\lambda = \begin{cases} (y^\lambda - 1)/\lambda & \text{if } \lambda \neq 0 \\ \log(y) & \text{if } \lambda = 0 \end{cases}$$

In Box-Cox transformation, λ can also be decimals, such as ½ or ¼, not necessarily being always integer. For Box-Cox transformation, log is not always the best transform. The best transformation can be decided by the degree and sign of skewness, which can be calculated using the stata command of 'boxcox'.

In application, the Box-Cox transformation of the outcome variable can make the residuals more approximate to normal distribution, thus reducing the problem caused by heteroscedasticity and kurtosis of the distribution of healthcare expenditure data and improving the precision and robustness of the estimation of the β_i hat. But the estimated β_i hat through the Box-Cox transformation, using either via OLS or maximum likelihood estimates, is related to the Box-Cox transformed y, such as log(y), but not the raw-scale value of y. In fact, no policy maker is interested in a transformed y, such as log(y). Researchers need to retransform back the estimates to raw-scale expenditure. Due to heteroscedasticity, retransforming back is not straightforward and may lead to a biased estimation of the raw-scale value of healthcare expenditure (Manning, 1998).

2.4.3.1.3 GLM

Developed in 1972 by Nelder and Wedderburn, GLMs are a synthesis and extension of common familiar regression models such as the linear models estimated through OLS and logit or probit models (Nelder and Wedderburn, 1972). GLM includes three parts:

1) the distribution of y, which is reflected through the mean-variance relationship, i.e. variance function. The distribution of y usually belongs to exponential family, such as normal, Binomial, Poisson, Gamma, or Inverse Gaussian distributions.
2) the linear part, which is a linear function of a set of predictors, $\eta = x_i\beta_i$.
3) a smooth and invertible linearizing link function g(.), which transforms the expectation of y, not the y in the raw-scale value, $\mu \equiv E(y|x)$, into the linear part $x_i\beta_i$:

$$g(\mu) = \eta = x_i\beta_i$$

A standard GLM assumes a specific link function to fit data distribution before the model converges. Some common link functions are listed in Table 2.5. The last two link functions, logit or probit, in Table 2.5 belong to binomial data. For healthcare expenditure data, the link function can be one of the first five options in Table 2.5 (Fox, 2008). The choice of link functions can be decided via the Box-cox test. The typical link function for healthcare expenditure data is the log transformation (Hill and Miller, 2010).

As to the distribution of y represented by the mean-variance function, it is can be expressed as bellow:

$$v(y) = k\mu^\sigma = \begin{cases} k & \textit{if } \sigma = 0, \text{ called Gaussian nonlinear least square distribution.} \\ k\mu & \textit{if } \sigma = 1, \text{ called Poisson distribution.} \\ k\mu^2 & \textit{if } \sigma = 2, \text{ called Gamma distribtution.} \\ k\mu^3 & \textit{if } \lambda = \sigma, \text{ called inverse Gaussian distribution.} \end{cases}$$

where different σ (0,1,2,3) represents the different distributions. k represents a constant or the proportion of v(y) to μ^σ. The determination of σ can be obtained through Park test (Park, 1966; Hardin and Hilbe, 2007).

Table 2.5: Common link functions for general linear model

Link	$\eta=g(\mu)$	$\mu=g^{-1}(\eta)$
Identity	M	H
Log	$Log(\mu)$	e^η
Inverse	μ^{-1}	η^{-1}
Inverse-square	μ^{-2}	$\eta^{-1/2}$
Square-root	$\sqrt{\mu}$	η^2
Logit	$Log(\mu/(1-\mu))$	$1/(1+e^{-\eta})$
Probit	$\Phi^{-1}(\mu)$	$\Phi(\eta)$

Source: Fox, 2008.

GLM accommodates skewness and heteroscedasticity through variance-weighting and transforming μ, the expectation of y, instead of y. Thus it can avoid the problem of retransformation and take into account the underlying distribution of the dependent variable (Wedderburn, 1974). GLM uses data to find distributional variance and link function. However, sometimes it is not always feasible to locate an appropriate variance or link function for GLM *a priori* using the separate tests of link and variance mentioned above. Improper specifications of link and variance functions could lead to a biased and inefficient estimation of β_i.

2.4.3.1.4 EEE

EEE were developed in 2005 by Basu and are semi-parametric models, which are an extension of GLM (Basu and Rathouz, 2005). EEE include:

1) parametric models to relate the mean $\mu(y)$ to the variance $v(y)$ through the functions of:

$$v(y) = \varphi h(\mu) = \begin{cases} \theta_1 \mu^{\theta_2} & \text{, for power variance} \\ \theta_1 \mu + \theta_2 \mu^2, & \text{for quadratic variance} \end{cases}$$

where ϕ is the dispersion parameter and θ_1 as well as θ_2 decide which the distribution of y belongs to, such as Poisson, Gamma or Inverse Gaussian distributions.

2) a link function applying Box-Cox transformation which is governed by another parameter of λ as follows:

$$\eta = x_i \beta_i = g(\mu; \lambda) = \begin{cases} (\mu^\lambda - 1) / \lambda & \text{if } \lambda \neq 0 \\ \log(\mu) & \text{if } \lambda = 0 \end{cases}$$

Thus, the variance function of EEE is $h(\mu; \theta_1, \theta_2)$ and the link function of EEE is $g(\mu; \lambda)$. Via extended quasi-likelihood estimation, β_i's are calculated together with θ_1, θ_2, and λ for EEE (Basu and Rathouz, 2005; Hill and Miller, 2010).

Comparing GLM and EEE, one can summarize that EEE are different from GLM in three aspects. First, the link and variance functions for GLM are set and fixed by researchers *a priori*, i.e. before the model converges and prior to the estimation of β_i's coming out. While in EEE, the link and variance functions are flexible and they do not need to be judged before the model converges. Thus EEE can fit the data into the best link and variance functions and is especially useful and offer robust estimates when no specific distribution of the outcome variable can be set by investigators before the model converges. Second, EEE provide a richer class of variance functions so that they can accommodate data with skewness and heteroscedasticity better than GLM. Third, EEE estimate the link and variance functions at the same time, which is more efficiently than GLM which chooses link and variance functions separately.

However, EEE also have their limitations. On a practical level, EEE work best in analyses with larger sample sizes, i.e. N > 5,000. With a small sample size, EEE usually do not converge (Basu and Rathouz, 2005).

2.4.3.2 Multi-part modelling

The above single-equation models assume a single relationship between healthcare expenditure data and explanatory variables using one functional form. Actually, different parts of the healthcare expenditure data can have various responses to explanatory variables by using different functions for each part (Basu and Manning, 2009).

2.4.3.2.1 Two-part model

The most common practice of multi-part modelling is the two-part model where the possibility of incurring any healthcare expenditure is modelled separately from the magnitude of healthcare expenditure, given that some expenditure is incurred in the first place. This modelling option fits well the distribution of healthcare expenditure data with massive zero (Deb *et al.*, 2006; Hill and Miller, 2010). The two-part model is based on the logic that any non-negative random dependent variable y can be expressed as following:

$$E(y|x) = Pr(y > 0 \mid x)E(y \mid y > 0, x)$$

where $Pr(y>0|x)$ represents the probability of incurring any healthcare expenditure and is estimated by logit or probit model using the full sample and $E(y|y>0,x)$ represents the level of healthcare expenditure and is estimated by OLS, log(y), GLM, or EEE using observations with positive healthcare expenditure data only (Belotti *et al.*, 2012).

2.4.3.2.2 An extension of two-part model

Other researchers have come up with a four part model, an extension of the two-part model developed in the 1980s. They found that the highest values in healthcare expenditure made the whole expenditure data depart from log normality in the right-most tail and such non-log normality occurred mostly in inpatient expenditure, but not in outpatient expenditure. Thus, they separated data according to three types: non-spenders, outpatient-only spenders, and spenders with inpatient utilization. In each part, they calculated the probability and expectation of positive expenditure. In this way, they analyzed the patterns and determinants of healthcare expenditure in a more detailed and accurate manner than the single two-part model (Duan et al., 1983).

This method is different from the one that uses two two-part models that separately model outpatient and inpatient care because those use inpatient care are likely to use outpatient care within a fixed recall period as well, making the two-part model for inpatient care not independent from the two-part model for out-patient care (Duan et al., 1983).

2.4.3.2.3 A generalized version of multi-part model

Based on the studies by other researchers (Efron, 1988; Donald et al., 2000), Gilleskie and Mroz established a generalized version of the multi-part model, whose main logic is that the range of healthcare expenditure data can be separated into several different parts. This allows one to address the skewness of healthcare expenditure data. The expectation of the whole outcome variable equals the possibility of the outcome variable being in a specific part, represented by the linear function of $x_i\beta_j$, times the conditional means on being in each part. For those healthcare expenditure data with only positive observations, it is best to opt for equal widths in each part. For those healthcare expenditure data with 0 observations, 0 observations can be in one single part and the rest can be put in the remaining parts in which an equal number of positive expenditures locate. If healthcare expenditure data is broken into more than two parts, the dataset needs a relatively large sample size to allow the model to converge (Gilleskie and Mroz, 2004).

In summary, every model of analyzing healthcare expenditure data listed above has its own advantages and disadvantages. The most appropriate model is the one that considers the nature and distribution of expenditure data (Basu and Manning, 2009).

2.4.4 The model that I chose to analyze OOP expenditure in this study

My analytical model chosen for OOP expenditure was based on the nature and distribution of my expenditure data (Basu and Manning, 2009), which had two characteristics.

First, they contained a massive amount of zero expenditure observations. This was due to a high proportion of individuals who either did not use any health services (non-users) or used services without having to pay anything OOP within the free health care system in Malawi. Thus, the model that I chose for OOP expenditure could accommodate data with massive zero observations. Considering that non-spenders might have a different relationship with covariates from those spenders (Basu and Manning, 2009), multi-part modelling was more feasible than single-equation modelling to deal with data with massive observations with zero. To take my relatively small sample size into account, I preferred a two-part model to a multi-part model with more than two parts for my expenditure analysis.

Figure 2.2: Kernel density estimate of raw healthcare expenditure data in my analysis.

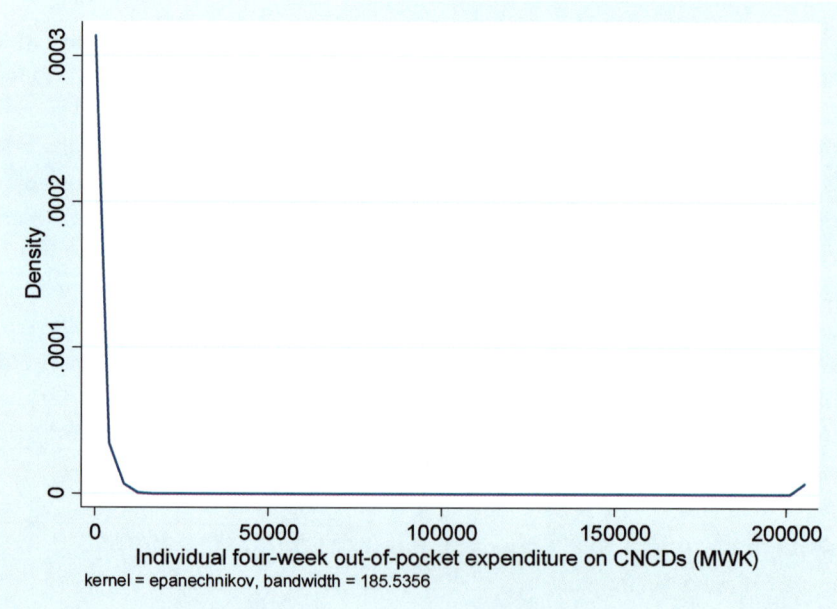

For the two-part model, how to model the first-part is relatively fixed, either logit or probit, while how to model the second-part needs to consider the distribution of the positive healthcare expenditure data. The available options for the second-part in a two-part model are OLS, Box-Cox transformation, GLM, and EEE (Basu and Manning, 2009). The positive healthcare expenditure data in my study contained a heavy right tail (Figure 2.2). Thus, OLS was not a proper option for the second-part in the two-part model since it might lead to a biased estimation in this case (Fu *et al.*, 2011). Due to re-transformation problems (Manning, 1998), the Box-Cox transformation was not a suitable option for my study either. Considering that EEE require a large dataset (Basu and Rathouz, 2005), EEE were not an applicable option in my study either. GLM is another option to correct skewness and heteroscedasticity when it can specify the link and variance functions *in priori* using some tests (Wedderburn, 1974). To identify link function, I used the Stata command of 'boxcox'. The test showed that I could not reject the hypothesis that the link function was log (p=0.109) but I could reject other forms of link functions, such as identity, inverse, inverse square (all $p<0.05$). Graphically, the log transformed positive healthcare expenditure data in my analysis reduced skewness and kurtosis from raw data greatly and showed improved symmetry (Figure 2.3). So I chose log transformation as the link function. To identify variance function, I used the Park test (Park, 1966; Hardin and Hilbe, 2007). The result revealed that I could not reject the hypothesis that the positive healthcare expenditure in my analysis belonged to Inverse Gaussian distribution (p=0.1038) but I could reject other variance functions, such as Gaussian nonlinear least square distribution, Poisson distribution, and Gamma distribution (all $p<0.05$). So I chose Inverse Gaussian distribution as the variance function.

Figure 2.3: Kernel density estimate of log transformed healthcare expenditure data in my analysis.

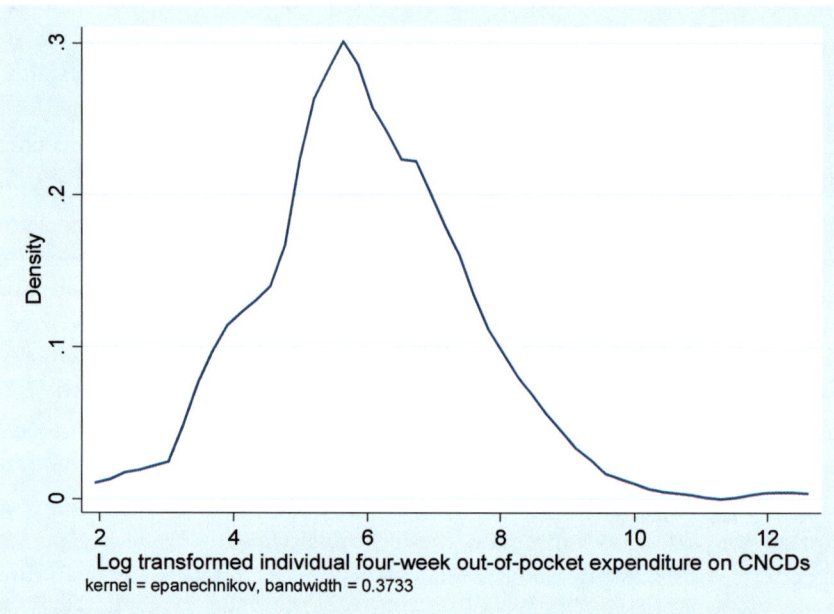

Considering the above two features of OOP expenditure on CNCDs in my analysis, I therefore decided to use a two-part model and specifically chose the GLM for the second-part to analyze my healthcare expenditure data. This approach is in line with other studies on determinants of healthcare expenditure (Matsaganis *et al.*, 2009; Schwarzkopf *et al.*, 2012).

2.5 Statistical analysis

2.5.1 Descriptive analysis for health seeking behavior

I used descriptive statistics to outline reported CNCDs and related patterns of health seeking. I conducted univariate and bivariate analyses to describe the frequency with which specific CNCDs were reported as well as their mean duration and perceived severity. I used the t-test to initially test differences in continuous explanatory variables (e.g.: age, disease duration, etc.) in subgroups disaggregating by health seeking options. In addition,

I performed the chi-square test to initially explore the difference of categorical explanatory variables (e.g.: sex, ethnicity, etc.) is subgroups disaggregating by health seeking options. Mean, standard deviation, and median were used to describe related household OOP expenditure on CNCDs.

2.5.2 Analytical analysis for health seeking behavior

As mentioned before, this study used MNL to confirm the associations detected by the bivariate analysis between a selected set of explanatory variables and health seeking choices. The MNL model in this study can be expressed as follows:

$$\text{Prob}(Y = 0) = \frac{1}{1 + e^{x\beta^0} + e^{x\beta^1}}$$

$$\text{Prob}(Y = 1) = \frac{e^{x\beta^0}}{1 + e^{x\beta^0} + e^{x\beta^1}}$$

$$\text{Prob}(Y = 2) = \frac{e^{x\beta^1}}{1 + e^{x\beta^0} + e^{x\beta^1}}$$

Y represents the outcome category of the various health seeking choices, where 'Y=0' is no care, 'Y=1' is informal care, 'Y=2' is formal care. β^0 and β^1 are a set of coefficients for each outcome category. X represents a set of explanatory variables. I used 'no care' as reference category (Table 2.2).

I checked the goodness-of-fit of the model using the Hosmer-Lemeshow test and computed robust standard errors to account for intra-household correlation.

In line with the literature on health seeking behavior not related to CNCDs, I expected that being a household head and Alomwe, higher education level of the household head, higher SES, lower proportion of people with CNCDs in a household (accounting for less competition on the intra-household allocation of resources), shorter distance to a health care facility, and higher severity of disease would all increase utilization of formal care. While being a household head and Alomwe, higher education level of the household head, higher SES, lower proportion of people with CNCDs in a household, and higher severity of disease would all increase utilization of informal care. Furthermore, based on clinical considerations, I expected individuals who suffered from "early detectable CNCDs" to make greater use of formal care, while individuals who suffered from "established CNCDs" to make greater use of informal care, given that their conditions are not an explicit target of the current EHP screening program (Table 2.2).

2.5.3 Descriptive analysis for OOP expenditure

I used descriptive statistics (mean and standard deviation) to outline the characteristics of the individuals in my sample who reported at least one CNCD and to compare respondents who incurred OOP expenditure to respondents who did not. I used the Spearman rank correlation test to explore the bivariate relationship between positive OOP expenditure and continuous explanatory variables (e.g.: age, disease duration) and the Wilcoxon rank-sum test to explore differences in positive OOP expenditure in subgroups defined by categorical variables (e.g.: sex, ethnicity, etc.).

In line with prior studies (Dror *et al.*, 2008; Rahman *et al.*, 2013), in order to explore the financial burden that OOP expenditure on CNCDs bears across SES quartiles, I calculated the OOP expenditure intensity ratio by dividing the four-week individual OOP expenditure on CNCDs by the four-week per capita household expenditure. Due to the skewness of this ratio, I used trimmed means to measure its tendency and Kruskal-Wallis test to analyze its distribution across SES quartiles.

In addition, the incidence of catastrophic spending due to CNCDs was computed as the proportion of households incurring catastrophic spending in relation to the total number of households reporting CNCDs (O'Donnell *et al.*, 2007; Engelgau *et al.*, 2012). I also analyzed the distribution of the incidence of catastrophic spending across SES quartiles. The incidence of impoverishment due to CNCDs was calculated in a similar way, i.e. the proportion of households being impoverished in relation to the total number of households reporting CNCDs (O'Donnell *et al.*, 2007; Engelgau *et al.*, 2012).

2.5.4 Analytical analysis for OOP expenditure

To construct the two-part model, I used data from all those who reported at least one CNCD without relying on trimmed data as I did for the descriptive analysis since GLM allows for skewness and heterogenerity (Wedderburn, 1974). The first-part, which relies on logistic regression to estimate the probability of incurred positive OOP expenditure, can be expressed as:

$$\ln\left[\frac{\text{Prob}(y>0\,|\,x)}{1-\text{Prob}(y>0\,|\,x)}\right] = \alpha + \sum \beta_i x_i$$

where y represents the outcome variable OOP expenditure on CNCDs, x_i represents a set of explanatory variables, β_i denotes coefficients of the corresponding estimates, α is constant.

The second-part of the model, which relies on the GLM with a log link to estimate the determinants of the amount of OOP expenditure, can be expressed as:

$$\ln\left(E(y|x)\right) = \alpha + \sum \beta_i x_i$$

where E(y) represents the expected value of the outcome variable. Other variables share similar notations from the first-part model.

I computed the model using the newly developed Stata command of tpm (Belotti *et al.*, 2012). Consistent with a prior study (Okunade *et al.*, 2010), I also estimated income elasticity from the second-part (expenditure level) model using the Stata command of margins.

In line with the literature on OOP expenditure on general conditions, I expected that being a household head and Alomwe, higher education level of the household head, higher SES, lower proportion of people with CNCDs in a household, and higher severity of disease would all increase the possibility of incurring and the level of OOP expenditure for CNCDs. Furthermore, to take the Malawian context into consideration, I hypothesized that people suffer from CNCDs targeted by screening programs through the EHP are less likely to incur OOP expenditure and high OOP expenditure for CNCDs (Table 2.2).

3. Results

3.1 General characteristics of the whole sample of the panel and respondents reporting a CNCD

Table 3.1 presents the characteristics of the complete sample of the panel as well as of the subsample reporting a CNCD. The panel included 5643 individuals from 1199 households. Out of 5643 individuals, 21.2% were the household head, 52.2% were female, and 77.6% were from Chiradzulu. Out of all respondents, 69.2% were Alomwe, 13.3% were Ayao, 7.9% were Angoni, and 4.0% were Anyanja. The respondents were young with the mean age being 21.4 years (standard deviation (SD) = 17.93). 47.4% of all respondents were under the age of 14. The mean six-month per capita household expenditure was approximately 29,720 MWK (SD = 70,310). The vast majority (81.1%) of all respondents lived in the household with a literate household head. The mean distance to nearest facilities was 2.30 km (SD = 1.30). The mean household size was 5.49 (SD = 1.95). The average number of children per household was 2.92 (SD = 1.42). The mean child/ adult ratio was 1.27 (SD = 0.86).

475 individuals (equivalent to 8.42% of all respondents) reporting at least one CNCD constitute the sample for my specific study. On average, compared with those not reporting any conditions related to CNCD, respondents who reported a CNCD were older, wealthier, and more likely to be household heads (Table 3.1). Still, 134 out of 475 (28.2%) individuals suffering from a CNCD were children below the age of 14. Among those reporting a CNCD, 269 (56.6%) were women and 206 (43.4%) were men. The average duration of CNCDs was 8.70 years (SD = 9.98). Out of 475 individuals reporting a CNCD, 59.2% perceived their condition as severe (i.e. to limit their daily activities), 17.7% suffered from a CNCD targeted through active screening programs by EHP, and 35.0% were from households with 50% or more household members reporting a CNCD (Table 3.1). Higher age, being female and household head, and perceiving their illness as serious were found to be positively associated with suffering from a CNCD targeted through active screening programs by EHP ($p < 0.0001$, $p < 0.01$, and $p < 0.0001$, and $p < 0.05$ respectively). Duration of disease was

found to be negatively associated with suffering from a CNCD targeted through active screening programs by EHP (p<0.01). No remarkable difference between individuals with a CNCD targeted through active screening programs by EHP and individuals with a CNCD not targeted by such programs was observed with regard to whether a person's ethnicity was Alomwe and household SES (Table 3.2).

Table 3.1: Description of the sample

	Entire sample		CNCD sample	
	(N=5643)		(N=475)	
	Mean	SD	Mean	SD
Age (years)	21.40	17.93	33.24	23.45
Six-month per capita household expenditure (MWK 1000)	29.72	70.31	47.92	139.31
Distance to nearest health facility (km)	2.30	1.30	2.26	1.31
Duration of diseases (years)	–	–	8.70	9.98
Household size (members)	5.49	1.95	5.17	2.03
	N	%	N	%
Being household head				
Yes	1198	21.2	147	31.0
No	4445	78.8	328	69.1
Sex				
Female	2945	52.2	269	56.6
Male	2698	47.8	206	43.4
Ethnicity				
Alomwe	3907	69.2	295	62.1
Other	1736	30.8	180	37.9
Household head literacy				
Yes	4575	81.1	381	80.2
No	1068	18.9	94	19.8
Household with 50% or more household members reporting a CNCD				
Yes	–	–	166	35.0
No	–	–	309	65.1

	Entire sample (N=5643)		CNCD sample (N=475)	
	Mean	SD	Mean	SD
Perceiving a CNCD as serious				
Yes	–	–	281	59.2
No	–	–	194	40.8
CNCDs targeted by screening program				
Yes	–	–	84	17.7
No	–	–	391	82.3

Table 3.2: Age, sex, being household head and Alomwe, duration, perceived severity, and household SES by CNCDs classification

	Early detectable CNCDs (n=84)		Established CNCDs (n=391)		
	Mean	SD	Mean	SD	P-value
Age (years)	45.57	15.75	30.59	24.00	<0.0001 [a]
Being female (%)	70.24	46.00	53.71	49.93	0.0060 [b]
Being the household head (%)	51.19	50.29	26.60	44.24	<0.0001 [b]
Being Alomwe (%)	65.48	47.83	61.38	48.75	0.4830 [b]
Duration (years)	5.63	5.97	9.36	10.53	0.0018 [a]
Perceived severity (%)	70.24	46.00	56.78	49.60	0.023 [b]
Six-month per capita household expenditure (MWK 1000)	56.90	184.35	46.00	127.81	0.5155 [a]

Notes: SES = social-economic status, [a] t-test, [b] chi-square test.

A total of 515 conditions were reported by these 475 respondents (Table 3.3). Out of 475 respondents reporting CNCDs, 428 (90.1%) reported only one CNCD, 43 (9.1%) reported two CNCDs, and 4 (0.8%) reported three CNCDs. The mean age of those suffering from only one CNCD and more than one CNCD was 31.86 years (SD = 22.78) and 45.79 years (SD = 25.86) respectively. Out of 515 conditions, the three most frequently reported CNCDs were chronic musculoskeletal conditions & chronic pain syndromes (n=126, accounting for 24.5% of all reported conditions), chronic respiratory conditions (n=98, 19.0%), and chronic cardiovascular conditions (n=95, 18.4%) (Table 3.3). Among individuals suffering from the three most frequently reported CNCDs, respondents reporting chronic musculoskeletal conditions & chronic pain syndromes were more likely to be with longer duration of disease, perceive their conditions as severe, and be from a less wealthy household than respondents reporting chronic respiratory and chronic cardiovascular conditions; respondents reporting chronic respiratory conditions were more likely to be younger and wealthier and were less likely to be female and the household head than respondents reporting chronic musculoskeletal conditions & chronic pain syndromes and chronic cardiovascular conditions; respondents reporting chronic cardiovascular conditions were more likely to be older, female, the household head, and with shorter duration of diseases than respondents reporting chronic musculoskeletal conditions & chronic pain syndromes and chronic respiratory conditions (Table 3.4).

Table 3.3: Reported cases of CNCDs

Reported cases per each CNCD category	N	%
Chronic musculoskeletal conditions & chronic pain syndromes	126	24.5
Chronic respiratory conditions	98	19.0
Chronic cardiovascular conditions	95	18.4
Chronic sense organ conditions	65	12.6
Chronic neuropsychiatric conditions	47	9.1
Chronic digestive conditions	42	8.2
Chronic skin or oral conditions	27	5.2
Malignant neoplastic conditions	6	1.2
Chronic genitourinary conditions	4	0.8
Other chronic problems	3	0.6
Chronic endocrine conditions	2	0.4
Total	515	100

Table 3.4: Age, sex, being household head and Alomwe, duration, perceived severity, and household SES by the three most frequently reported CNCDs

	chronic pain (n=126)		chronic respiratory diseases (n=98)		cardiovascular diseases (n=95)	
	Mean	SD	Mean	SD	Mean	SD
Age (years)	45.71	22.18	19.57	20.72	48.16	17.88
Being female (%)	61.90	48.76	46.94	50.16	72.63	44.82
Being the household head (%)	42.86	49.68	15.31	36.19	47.87	50.22
Being Alomwe (%)	59.52	49.28	56.12	49.88	63.16	48.49
Duration (years)	10.94	13.38	8.48	9.09	7.25	9.08
Perceived severity (%)	69.05	46.41	54.08	50.09	67.37	47.14
Six-month per capita household expenditure (MWK 1000)	39.69	69.90	58.69	173.67	57.58	175.00

Note: SES = social-economic status.

3.2 Descriptive statistics for health seeking behavior on CNCDs

Out of 475 individuals who reported at least one CNCD, 177 (37.3%) did not seek any care, 298 sought some form of care, either formal or informal. Out of those who sought care, 202 (67.8%) sought formal care, 96 (32.2%) sought informal care. Among those who sought informal care, 31 (32.3%) visited a traditional healer, and 65 (67.7%) resorted to home treatment. 182 out of 202 (90.1%) of those seeking formal care chose public facilities.

Out of 126 individuals reporting chronic musculoskeletal conditions & chronic pain syndromes, 55 (43.7%) sought formal care, 35 (27.8%) sought informal care, and 36 (28.6%) sought no care. Out of 98 individuals reporting chronic respiratory conditions, 37 (37.8%) used formal care, 19 (19.4%) used informal care, and 42 (42.9%) did nothing for their condition. Out of 95 individuals reporting chronic cardiovascular conditions, 49 (51.6%) chose formal care, 12 (12.6%) chose informal care, and 34 (38.8%) chose no care.

Table 3.5: Characteristics of sub-groups disaggregated by health seeking options

	No care (N=177)		Formal care (N=202)		Informal care (N=96)		p-value[a] (1)vs(2)	p-value[a] (1)vs(3)
	Mean	SD	Mean	SD	Mean	SD		
Age (years)	30.64	22.51	35.54	23.96	33.16	23.79	0.0417	0.3889
Six-month per capita household expenditure (MWK 1000)	37.16	53.02	56.64	196.54	49.42	97.58	0.2020	0.1794
Distance to nearest health facility (km)	2.26	1.28	2.29	1.36	2.18	1.26	0.7974	0.6380
Duration of diseases (years)	9.42	10.20	7.59	8.46	9.71	12.15	0.0569	0.8328
Household size (members)	5.31	1.99	5.08	2.05	5.15	2.07	0.2730	0.5560
	N	%	N	%	N	%	p-value[b] (1)vs(2)	p-value[b] (1)vs(3)
Being household head								
Yes	39	22.0	73	36.1	35	36.5	0.003	0.010
No	138	78.0	129	63.9	61	63.5		
Sex								
Female	107	60.5	115	56.9	47	49.0	0.487	0.067
Male	70	39.5	87	43.1	49	51.0		
Ethnicity								
Alomwe	107	60.5	127	62.9	61	63.5		

	No care (N=177) (1)		Formal care (N=202) (2)		Informal care (N=96) (3)		p-value [a] (1)vs(2)	p-value [a] (1)vs(3)
	Mean	SD	Mean	SD	Mean	SD		
Other	70	39.5	75	37.1	35	36.5	0.629	0.616
Household head literacy								
Yes	142	80.2	162	80.2	77	80.2		
No	35	19.8	40	19.8	19	19.8	0.995	0.997
Household with 50% or more household members reporting a CNCD								
Yes	67	37.9	69	34.2	30	31.3		
No	110	62.1	133	65.8	66	68.8	0.454	0.276
Perceiving a CNCD as serious								
Yes	73	41.2	156	77.2	52	54.2		
No	104	58.8	46	22.8	44	45.8	<0.001	0.041
CNCDs targeted by screening program								
Yes	29	16.4	48	23.8	7	7.3		
No	148	83.6	154	76.2	89	92.7	0.075	0.034

Notes: [a] P-value is for t-test, which was used to initially test differences in continuous explanatory variables (e.g.: age, disease duration, etc.) in subgroups disaggregating by health seeking options.

[b] P-value is for chi-square test, which was used to initially explore the difference of categorical explanatory variables (e.g.: sex, ethnicity, etc.) are subgroups disaggregating by health seeking options.

Table 3.5 presents the comparison of the three sub-groups disaggregated by health seeking options, i.e. no care, formal care, and informal care. On average, compared with those who did not seek any care for their condition, respondents who chose formal and informal care were both more likely to be older, wealthier, male, Alomwe and the household head, as well as perceive their CNCDs as severe and were both less likely to be from households with 50% or more household members reporting a CNCD. In addition, individuals who opted for formal care for their chronic condition were more likely to be older, wealthier, with shorter duration of the disease, perceive their CNCD as serious and suffer from a CNCD targeted through active screening programs by EHP than the other two sub-groups of people, i.e. those seeking informal care and those seeking no care. Individuals who chose informal care to treat CNCDs were less likely to be female, from households with 50% or more household members reporting a CNCD, and suffer from a CNCD targeted through active screening programs by EHP than the other two sub-groups of people, i.e. those seeking formal care and those seeking no care.

Through bivariate analysis, I identified quite a number of factors that correlated with health seeking behavior. When comparing formal care with no care, higher age, shorter duration, being the household head, higher perceived severity, and CNCDs targeted by screening program were positively associated with the use of formal care ($p<0.05$, $p<0.10$, $p<0.01$, $p<0.001$, and $p<0.10$ respectively). No remarkable difference between individuals choosing formal care and no care was observed with regard to household SES, distance to nearest health facility, household size, being female and Alomwe, household head literacy, and proportion of people with CNCDs within the household. When comparing informal care with no care, being the household head, higher perceived severity, and CNCDs not targeted by screening program were positively associated with the use of informal care (all $p<0.05$). Being female was found to be negatively associated with use of informal care, though the significance level was set at the 10% level. No remarkable difference between individuals choosing informal care and no care was observed with regard to age, household SES, distance to nearest health facility, duration of disease, household size, being Alomwe, household head literacy, and proportion of people with CNCDs within the household (Table 3.5).

3.3 Analytical results for health seeking behavior on CNCDs

Table 3.6 reports results from the MNL model. The MNL model passed the test of Hosmer-Lemeshow (p>0.05), identifying that the MNL model I used fit well for the set of observations in this study. Contrary to the bivariate analysis, after controlling for confounders, I found only a few factors that associated with health seeking options. In the model of formal care versus no care, I found that higher SES, being a household head, and higher perceived severity significantly increased the probability of using formal care (for these three explanatory variables, p<0.01). Longer illness duration and the proportion of people with CNCDs in a household were negatively associated with formal care utilization (p<0.01 and p<0.1 respectively). Similarly, in the model of informal care versus no care, I found that higher SES, being a household head, and higher perceived severity significantly increased the probability of using informal care (p<0.05, p<0.05, and p<0.01 respectively). Suffering from "early detectable CNCDs" and the proportion of people with CNCDs in a household were negatively associated with informal care utilization (p<0.01 and p<0.1 respectively).

Table 3.6: Health seeking behavior: Estimated coefficients in multinomial logit model

	Formal care vs. No-care			Informal care vs. No-care		
	coef	Robust s.e.[a]	p-value	coef	Robust s.e.[a]	p-value
Intercept	-1.378***	0.483	0.004	-1.055**	0.529	0.046
Age	0.006	0.006	0.337	0.004	0.008	0.592
Being the household head	0.919***	0.316	0.004	0.941**	0.393	0.017
Sex	0.012	0.254	0.961	-0.186	0.311	0.550
Ethnicity	0.206	0.237	0.386	0.200	0.292	0.494
Household head literacy	0.378	0.299	0.206	0.256	0.315	0.417
Six-month per capita household expenditure	0.003***	0.001	0.005	0.003**	0.001	0.046

	Formal care vs. No-care			Informal care vs. No-care		
	coef	Robust s.e.[a]	p-value	coef	Robust s.e.[a]	p-value
Household with 50% or more household members reporting a CNCD	-0.444*	0.256	0.083	-0.556*	0.320	0.082
Distance to nearest facilities	-0.037	0.092	0.688	-0.074	0.101	0.465
Duration of CNCDs	-0.040***	0.012	0.001	-0.017	0.014	0.242
Perceived severity	1.819***	0.247	<0.001	0.791***	0.273	0.004
CNCDs targeted by screening program	-0.241	0.308	0.434	-1.423***	0.489	0.004
Pseudo R^2 = 0.1025; Wald	$\chi^2(22) = 89.69, P > \chi^2 = 0.0000$					
Hosmer-Lemeshow (goodness of fit) test	$\chi^2(16) = 12.497, P > \chi^2 = 0.709$					

Notes: [a] Robust Standard errors adjusted for household clusters.

* $p<0.1$, ** $p< 0.05$, *** $p< 0.01$.

3.4 Descriptive statistics for OOP expenditure on CNCDs

Figure 3.1 shows the overview of OOP expenditure on CNCDs in the study setting. Out of 298 respondents who sought care due to CNCDs, 102 (34.2%) did not incur any OOP expenditure. Together with 177 of those seeking no care, 279 out of 475 (58.7%) of those reporting at least one CNCD did not incur at any level of CNCD-related OOP expenditure in the four weeks prior to the survey date, while 196 (41.3%) did. Out of the 196 individuals who incurred OOP expenditure, 123 (62.8%) only incurred spending on medical care, not on transport.

Figure 3.1: Overview of OOP expenditure on CNCDs in rural Malawi.

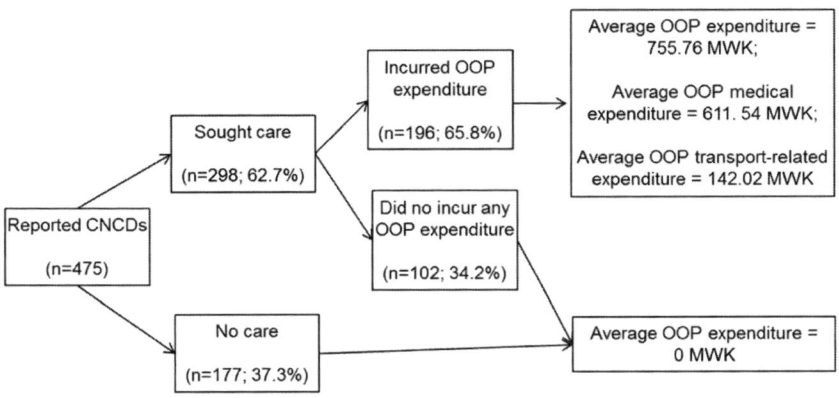

Notes: OOP = out-of pocket;
[a] The use of trimmed means implied losing 18 out of 196 observations for those incurring OOP expenditure on CNCDs.

The average OOP expenditure for those who paid for care related to CNCDs OOP was 755.76 MWK (SD = 1000.12), with 611.54 MWK (SD = 983.30) being paid on medical care and 142.02 MWK (SD = 247.38) on transportation (Figure 3.1). For those who used formal care, the average OOP expenditure on direct medical care and related travel was 632.38 MWK (SD = 1153.33) and 236.18 MWK (SD = 384.48) respectively. For those who used informal care, the average OOP expenditure on direct medical care and related travel was 601.58 MWK (SD = 843.28) and 55.79 MWK (SD = 155.48) respectively. In addition, for those reporting chronic musculoskeletal conditions & chronic pain syndromes, the average OOP expenditure on direct medical care and related travel was 390.74 MWK (SD = 606.86) and 75.37 MWK (SD = 152.62) respectively. For those reporting chronic respiratory conditions, the average OOP expenditure on direct medical care and related travel was 639.33 MWK (SD = 930.91) and 146.67 MWK (SD = 243.16) respectively. For those reporting chronic cardiovascular conditions, the average OOP expenditure on direct medical care and related travel was 1614.86 MWK (SD = 4129.22) and 382.97 MWK (SD = 839.57) respectively (Table 3.7).

Table 3.7: OOP medical and transport-related expenditures

	Medical expenditure (MWK)		Transportation expenditure (MWK)	
	Mean (SD)	median	Mean (SD)	median
Formal care (n=112) [a]	632.38 (1153.33)	200	236.18 (384.48)	100
Informal care (n=84) [a]	601.58 (843.28)	300	55.79 (155.48)	0
Total	611.54 (983.30)	250	142.02 (247.38)	0
Desegregated by the three most frequently reported CNCDs				
Chronic pains (n=60) [b]	390.74 (606.86)	215	75.37 (152.62)	0
Chronic respiratory conditions (n=32) [b]	639.33 (930.91)	225	146.67 (243.16)	0
Chronic cardiovascular conditions (n=39) [b]	1614.86 (4129.22)	250	382.97 (839.57)	150

Notes: OOP = out-of pocket.

[a] The use of trimmed means implied losing 10 out of 112 individuals having incurred an expenditure and having used formal care, and eight out of 84 having incurred an expenditure and having used informal care.

[b] The use of trimmed means implied losing six out of 60, two out of 32, and two out of 39 individuals having incurred an expenditure among individuals reporting chronic pains, chronic respiratory conditions, and chronic cardiovascular conditions respectively.

Table 3.8: Characteristics of sub-groups of individuals based on whether they incurred OOP expenditure

	Not incurring OOP expenditure (N=279)		Incurring OOP expenditure (N=196)		Spearman R [a]	p-value [c]
	Mean	SD	Mean	SD		
Individual OOP expenditure for CNCDs (MWK) [b]	–	–	755.76	1000.12	–	–
Age (years)	31.89	22.66	35.15	24.46	0.0945	0.1877
Duration of diseases (years)	8.63	9.53	8.81	10.61	0.0868	0.2266
Four-week per capita household expenditure (MWK 1000)	7.09	18.50	9.27	28.63	0.2359	0.0009
Proportion of people with CNCDs within the household	0.37	0.22	0.39	0.25	-0.0492	0.4939
Distance to nearest health facility (km)	2.28	1.26	2.22	1.38	-0.0233	0.7462

	Not incurring OOP expenditure (N=279)		Incurring OOP expenditure (N=196)		Spear-man R[a]	p-value[c]
	Mean	SD	Mean	SD		
Household size (members)	5.22	1.97	5.11	2.12	-0.0300	0.6758
	N	%	N	%	Mean (MWK)[b]	p-value[d]
Female						
Yes	169	60.6	100	51.0	671.61	
No	110	39.4	96	49.0	875.91	0.8106
Ethnicity						
Alomwe	174	62.4	121	61.7	933.62	
Other	105	37.6	75	38.3	524.06	0.2017
Being the household head						
Yes	74	26.5	73	37.2	788.66	
No	205	73.5	123	62.8	735.81	0.1247
Perceiving a CNCD as serious						
Yes	142	50.9	139	70.9	900.83	
No	137	49.1	57	29.1	587.92	0.1662
CNCDs targeted by EPH screening program						
Yes	53	19.0	31	15.8	2628.97	
No	226	81.0	165	84.2	651.58	0.0821
Household head literacy						
Yes	226	81.0	155	79.1	826.49	
No	53	19.0	41	20.9	566.49	0.5341
Use of formal care						
Yes	90	32.3	112	57.1	981.13	
No	189	67.7	84	42.9	578.16	0.0861

Notes: OOP = out-of pocket; SD = standard deviation.

[a] Spearman rank correlation was used to explore the relationship between positive OOP expenditure on CNCDs and continuous explanatory variables (e.g.: age, disease duration, etc.).

[b] Trimmed mean was used to depict OOP expenditure for CNCDs sample, those incurring OOP expenditure and different subgroups out of those incurring OOP expenditure. The use of trimmed mean implied losing 46 out of 475 for CNCDs sample and 18 out of 196 observations for both those incurring OOP expenditure and subgroups out of those incurring OOP expenditure.

[c] P-value is for Spearman rank correlation.

[d] P-value is for Wilcoxon rank-sum test, which was used to initially test differences in positive OOP expenditure in subgroups defined by categorical variables (e.g.: sex, ethnicity, etc.) based on 196 observations of those incurring OOP expenditure.

Table 3.8 presents the comparison of the two subgroups of individuals based on whether they incurred OOP expenditure on CNCDs or not. On average, compared with those who did not incur any OOP expenditure, individuals who incurred OOP expenditure were more likely to come from a wealthier household, be the household head, perceive their CNCD as severe, used formal healthcare services and were less likely to be female.

The right-most two columns of Table 3.8 present bivariate relationship between incurring positive OOP expenditure on CNCDs and its possible determinants. This study found that four-week per capita household expenditure was positively correlated with OOP expenditure (p=0.009). Suffering from an EHP-targeted CNCD and use of formal care were found to be positively associated with positive OOP expenditure on CNCDs (both p<0.1). No remarkable difference of positive OOP expenditure was observed with regard to age, duration of disease, proportion of people with CNCDs within the household, distance to nearest health facility, household size, being female, household head, Alomwe, perceiving CNCDs as serious, and household head literacy.

Table 3.9 shows the distribution of the OOP expenditure intensity ratio across SES quartiles. Those who incurred OOP expenditure spent on average the equivalent 22.0% of their monthly non-health expenditure on care related to CNCDs. This proportion differed significantly across SES quartiles (p<0.01), with the poorest households spending the highest proportion on care for CNCDs.

Table 3.9: OOP expenditure intensity ratio (ratio between OOP expenditure on CNCDs and four-week per capita household expenditure)

	Mean (SD)	Median	N
1st Quartile (lowest SES)	0.542 [a] (0.750)	0.303	42
2nd Quartile	0.300 [a] (0.488)	0.186	21
3rd Quartile	0.201 [a] (0.272)	0.092	58
4th Quartile (highest SES)	0.113 [a] (0.139)	0.052	75
Total	0.220 [a] (0.309)	0.098	196
Kruskal-Wallis	χ^2 =11.999	p=0.007	

Notes: OOP = out-of pocket.

[a] The use of trimmed means implied losing four out of 42, two out of 21, four out of 58, six out of 75 and 18 out of 196 individuals for households in 1st, 2nd, 3rd, 4th quartile and all those who incurred OOP expenditure respectively.

Table 3.10 presents the incidence of catastrophic spending due to CNCDs at the household level. Out of 244 households with at least one household member reporting a chronic non-communicable illness and seeking care for such a condition, 21.3% reported that direct costs due to their chronic illness exceeded 10% of household non-food expenditure. Increasing the threshold to 25% and 40% reduced the incidence of catastrophic spending to 10.7% and 4.5%, respectively. The incidence of catastrophic spending was different across SES quartiles with the poorest households being more likely to incur catastrophic spending due to CNCDs.

Table 3.11 presents household impoverishment due to CNCDs. Out of 244 households with at least one household member reporting a chronic non-communicable condition and seeking care for such a condition, 43.0% already lived under the international poverty line of $1.25 per person per day before expenses in form of any direct out-of-pocket payment due to CNCDs occurred. Once adjusted for spending on care for CNCDs, impoverishment increased to 44.7% in respect to the international poverty line.

Table 3.10: Incidence of household catastrophic spending due to CNCDs (n=244)

	10%	25%	40%
1st Quartile (lowest SES) (n=51)	35.3%	23.5%	9.8%
2nd Quartile (n=44)	20.5%	11.4%	4.5%
3rd Quartile (n=65)	23.1%	7.7%	3.1%
4th Quartile (highest SES) (n=84)	11.9%	4.8%	2.4%
Total (n=244)	21.3%	10.7%	4.5%

Table 3.11: Household impoverishment due to CNCDs (n=244)

Pre-payment poverty rate	Post-payment poverty rate
43.0%	44.7%

3.5 Analytical results for OOP expenditure on CNCDs

Table 3.12 shows the results of the two-part model. In the first-part of the logistic regression model, I found that higher perceived disease severity and use of formal care were significantly associated with an increased likelihood of incurring OOP expenditure on CNCDs (both p<0.001). Suffering from a

CNCD targeted by EHP screening was negatively associated with the possibility of incurring OOP expenditure ($p < 0.05$). In the second-part GLM, I found that being female, Alomwe, the household head, longer duration of disease, suffering from a CNCD targeted by EHP screening, higher SES, household head literacy, and use of formal care were all positively associated with the amount of OOP expenditure on CNCDs ($p < 0.001$, $p < 0.01$, $p < 0.01$, $p < 0.05$, $p < 0.05$, $p < 0.05$, $p < 0.05$, and $p < 0.01$ respectively). The proportion of people with CNCDs living in a household was negatively associated with the amount of OOP expenditure on CNCDs ($p < 0.01$).

In addition, income elasticity, estimated from the second-part GLM in two-part model, at the mean and median of four-week per capita household expenditure was calculated as 0.0494 and 0.0233 respectively. Average income elasticity for the 196 observations of those incurring OOP expenditure on CNCDs was 0.0475.

Table 3.12: Two-part model for determinants of OOP expenditure on CNCDs (first-part: logit model, second-part: generalized linear model with log link and inverse Gaussian distribution)

	First part: probability of positive OOP expenditure (n=279)			Second part: determinants of the amount of OOP expenditure (n=196)		
	OR	95% CI	p-value	Coeff	95% CI	p-value
Age	1.003	0.992, 1.015	0.560	0.004	-0.015, 0.023	0.682
Female	0.720	0.464, 1.112	0.143	1.364***	0.589, 2.138	0.001
Alomwe	1.023	0.686, 1.526	0.910	0.969**	0.311, 1.626	0.004
Being the household head	1.468	0.850, 2.536	0.169	1.709**	0.591, 2.826	0.003
Duration of CNCDs	0.996	0.975, 1.017	0.683	0.027*	0.006, 0.049	0.013
Perceiving CNCD as serious	2.070**	1.341, 3.195	0.001	0.775	-0.151, 1.700	0.101
CNCDs targeted by EHP screening program	0.525*	0.296, 0.932	0.028	0.942*	0.140, 1.744	0.021
Four-week per capita household expenditure	1.004	0.992, 1.015	0.533	0.004*	0.0001, 0.008	0.042
Household head being literate	0.963	0.588, 1.577	0.882	0.897*	0.063, 1.731	0.035
Proportion of people with CNCDs within the household	1.186	0.483, 2.912	0.709	-3.184**	-5.107, -1.261	0.001
Use of formal care	2.376***	1.569, 3.598	0.000	1.033***	0.432, 1.635	0.001
Distance to nearest health facility	0.919	0.793, 1.064	0.259	-0.067	-0.392, 0.257	0.685

Notes: OOP = out-of pocket; OR = odds ratio; CI = confidence interval.
* p< 0.05, ** p<0.01, *** p<0.001.

4. Discussion

4.1 Disease categories and classification

This study explored behavior in relation to a broader spectrum of CNCDs than currently at the core of the WHO policy guidelines (World Health Organization, 2011a) on the major four health conditions (cancers, cardiovascular diseases, chronic respiratory diseases, diabetes), and related risk factors. The decision to look at a broader spectrum of CNCDs was purposeful and motivated by the need to fill a general knowledge void on health seeking and OOP expenditure practices, beyond the specific relevance of the single conditions. It has to be recognized that given its exclusive reliance on self-reported information, this study by no means aimed at assessing the accurate prevalence of CNCD.

In addition to the small number of cases in each disease category, the exclusive focus on health seeking and OOP expenditure in the process of health seeking motivated our decision to reclassify the 10 initial illness categories used to recall chronic symptoms and diseases during data collection into a simpler classification distinguishing only between two CNCD classes, "early detectable" vs. "established" CNCDs. As explained in the methods section, this simpler classification was not meant to replace clinically relevant classifications. It was rather expected to adequately reflect perceived need, as influenced by service availability in the Malawian context, and as such, be likely to shape health seeking. This classification allowed us to define a proxy for the motivation to seek healthcare driven either by the intention to prevent disease progression or by the intention to relieve or alleviate existing ailments.

4.2 Methodological considerations

4.2.1 Sample

The sample for this study was population-based, encompassing the rural population suffering from a wide range of CNCDs in Malawi. This is different from the majority of the limited existing studies on CNCDs in SSA relying on samples selected from patients with single CNCD in formal facilities.

Estimates of health seeking behavior and OOP expenditure obtained from a population-based study can account for the potential users of health care facilities and thus are more accurate in depicting people's treatment options and financial burden in relation to CNCDs (Akin *et al.*, 1995).

In spite of the efforts to obtain complete information by using both a disease classification and a list of symptoms, it is possible that in a generalized context of under diagnoses of CNCDs caused by poor health provision capacity from the supply side and limited awareness of preventing and controlling CNCDs from the demand side (Aspray *et al.*, 2000; Mbanya *et al.*, 2010), this study may underestimate the actual number of people living with CNCDs. This has probably constrained the effective sample size, limiting the ability to detect the effect of some variables on health seeking choices and OOP expenditure.

An indication that underreporting might have occurred comes from the fact that descriptive statistics indicated the existence of selection bias in CNCD reporting, with household heads and individuals who are older or wealthier reporting more conditions related to CNCDs than other respondents. The estimation of the effects should have ideally relied on a model that could account for potential, but not confirmed, selection bias (it cannot be excluded that higher reporting among certain groups simply reflects underlying prevalence of CNCDs in the study population). The structure of the data, however, did not allow this study to identify a suitable instrument and apply a Hausman selection model to the estimation of the parameters. This study therefore developed the model on the truncated sample of those reporting a CNCD in the first place, but reported descriptive statistics for the entire sample in line with prior studies (Gotsadze et al. 2005; Su and Flessa 2013; Dong et al. 2008). Thus, there could be differences between the overall sample and the truncated sample used for the analysis of healthcare seeking. The inability to confirm the existence and control for selection bias does not threaten the validity of the results *per se*, but indicates that the derived estimates could represent a lower end boundary of the true effect. Given the direction of the selection bias, SES and being a household head are likely to play a greater role in shaping health care decisions than what is observed in the model (Pokhrel *et al.*, 2010).

4.2.2 Data collection and data

The definition of CNCDs was straightforward, but included numerous and diverse conditions, which made it difficult to determine the exact limits of the different categories (Sridhar *et al.*, 2011). However, both disease categories and the underlying list used in this study were consistent with the existing literature on CNCDs (Gwatkin *et al.*, 1999; World Health Organization, 2008a; Nugent and Feigl, 2010), suggesting that hardly any better tool could have been used to elicit the recall of CNCD through means of a population-based survey (Kehoe *et al.*, 1994; Kriegsman *et al.*, 1996; Goldman *et al.*, 2003).

In line with what is frequently done for studies relying on self-reported morbidity (Van Minh *et al.*, 2008; Msyamboza *et al.*, 2011; Miszkurka *et al.*, 2012), this study used an approach that allowed us to transform, as accurately as possible, the information on chronic ailments perceived and reported by lay people into a commonly used CNCD categorization framework based on WHO criteria (World Health Organization, 2008a). It has to be recognized that this approach does not necessarily reflect the epidemiological burden of CNCDs among the study sample, as no clinical assessments were conducted to verify the reported illness information.

During data collection, interviewers conducted the face-to-face interviews in Chichewa, the local language in Malawi, while the questionnaire was first prepared in English by the team in University of Heidelberg. In spite of translating the questionnaire from English into Chichewa and then retranslating it into English and pre-testing it, one cannot rule out the possibility that the final questionnaire in Chichewa may lose a certain value of information compared to the original English version.

In addition, a few points regarding data need to be noted as well. First, in this study, information on OOP expenditure was collected based on the information reported directly by the individuals and may therefore be subject to recall bias. Like in many other rural settings in SSA, it was not possible for this study to validate the veridicity of the information provided by the respondents, given the absence of formal medical booklets documenting illness and healthcare seeking. The use of a four-week recall period, rather than a longer recall period as applied in other CNCD studies (Chuma *et al.*, 2007; Tharkar *et al.*, 2010; Huffman *et al.*, 2011; Guariguata *et al.*, 2012; Islam *et al.*, 2013), was designed to minimize recall bias (Merkesdal *et al.*, 2005; Islam *et al.*, 2013). Still, in line with prior research (Akweongo *et al.*, 2013; Atif *et al.*, 2014), I cannot exclude that in spite of the efforts to minimize recall bias, I did not to some extent underestimate or overestimate OOP expenditure. Underestimation of OOP expenditure might have occurred as the result of the fact that individuals may incur direct expenditure related to CNCD on larger time intervals and may have therefore not spent anything in the prior four weeks, because still in possession of enough medications to control their condition from a prior prescription (Yaffe *et al.*, 1978; Cohen and Carlson, 1994). On the contrary, overestimation of OOP expenditure might have occurred as a result of potential over-reporting the direct costs associated with health seeking due to CNCDs. Second, this study is based on cross-sectional data. Future analysis based on longitudinal data will be more suitable to establish causality in relation to factors shaping health seeking behavior and OOP expenditure on CNCDs. Third, due to problems regarding data availability in the study setting, this study only used the straight-line distance, not the actual route from people's home to the nearest facility, as the measure of distance to the nearest formal health care facility. However, in low-income countries the straight-line distance has been proved to be an adequate proxy of the actual route from people's home to the nearest facility for studies on health care utilization (Nesbitt *et al.*, 2014) .

4.2.3 Analytical approach

Being one of the first exploratory studies on determinants of health seeking behavior and OOP expenditure on CNCDs in SSA, this study used not only descriptive analysis but also the analytical model, controlling for confounders in the analysis. The analytical model of determinants of OOP expenditure needs further clarification. As explained in the methods section, this study included both non-users and users of health services without any OOP expenditure in the zero OOP expenditure group. This is based on the context of our study setting and our study perspective with a clear focus on individual OOP expenditure on CNCDs instead of the societal expenditure related to CNCDs. It should be emphasized here that individuals who used health care services related to CNCDs without incurring OOP expenditures are assumed to have consumed state-funded resources.

In addition, the methodology currently available to estimate catastrophic spending and impoverishment does not account for people who forego care, since these individuals do not report any out-of-pocket expenditure due to illness (O'Donnell *et al.*, 2007). Households forgoing treatment are usually the poorest in a community. Forgoing treatment causes further deterioration of one's health, often leading to further economic losses and deeper poverty. Thus, the real economic impact of CNCDs is likely to be much higher than what can be estimated using available methodology and what I was able to show in this study, using catastrophic spending and impoverishment as relevant indicators (O'Donnell *et al.*, 2007; Chuma and Maina, 2012).

4.3 Discussion of the results

4.3.1 Self-reported cases on CNCDs and characteristics of CNCD reporters

Though being inaccurate, studies relying on self-reported data still show certain information on characteristics of the prevalence of CNCDs as well as features of respondents reporting these conditions in SSA (Miszkurka *et al.*, 2012; Phaswana-Mafuya *et al.*, 2013) and in LMICs in general (Van Minh *et al.*, 2008; Amal *et al.*, 2011; Bhojani *et al.*, 2013). It is worthwhile to discuss self-reported cases and characteristics of CNCD reporters identified in this study.

First, the results in the dissertation showed relatively high levels of reported CNCD prevalence, with nearly one tenth of all respondents suffering from at least one CNCD. This study found that 18.4% of all conditions reported by 475 respondents (including children and adults) were chronic cardivascular conditions. The self-reported prevalence of chronic cardivascular conditions is similar to two other epidemiological studies in Malawi indicating that the prevalence of hypertension was about 33% and 23% of individuals aged 25–64 (Msyamboza *et al.*, 2011) and adults aged 18 and above (de Ramirez *et al.*, 2010) respectively. My dissertation also found that the most prevalent condition was chronic musculoskeletal conditions & chronic pain syndromes, accounting for 24.5% of all reported cases. The self-reported prevalence of the conditions is in line with one prevalence study of NCDs in Burkina Faso indicating that 24% of reported cases among adults aged 18 and above were back pain (Miszkurka *et al.*, 2012). The same study in Burkina Faso also found that the prevalence of asthma among adults was 11.6% (Miszkurka *et al.*, 2012), which is consistent with the self-reported prevalence of chronic respiratory conditions reported in this study. Second, this study confirmed the high prevalence of CNCDs, especially chronic respiratory conditions, among the very young population, which is consistent with other studies on disease burden due to CNCDs in SSA (Aït-Khaled *et al.*, 2001; Unwin *et al.*, 2001; Lopez *et al.*, 2006) and in LMICs (World Health Organization, 2011a). Third, more women than men were found to report CNCDs, which is similar to studies on CNCDs in other SSA countries (Tagoe, 2013) and from LMICs (Bhojani *et al.*, 2013; Uddin *et al.*, 2014). Fourth, those reporting a CNCD were found to be wealthier than those not reporting any of these conditions, which is in line with other evidence on general conditions in SSA (Dong *et al.*, 2008; Pokhrel *et al.*, 2010).

4.3.2 Options of health seeking behavior on CNCDs

This study found that over one third of respondents reporting a CNCD sought no care. The high proportion of seeking no care among individual reporting CNCDs is consistent with findings on health seeking behavior on CNCDs from other countries in SSA (Chuma *et al.*, 2007; Goudge *et al.*, 2009a; Faronbi *et al.*, 2014) and in LMICs (Baliga *et al.*, 2013; Uddin *et al.*, 2014). In the context of Malawi, where health care services are in principle provided free of charge at point of use, this result appears even more striking and suggests the existence of barriers to access related to care for CNCDs. It needs to be noted, however, that given the limited recall period, it cannot be excluded that those not reporting any health care utilization were individuals who would seek care at other points in time.

The analysis also revealed that a bit more than 30% of those reporting having suffered from CNCDs chose to utilize formal care, which is pursuant to two other population-based studies indicating that about one third of those reporting CNCDs (Lopes Ibanez-Gonzalez and Norris, 2013) and chronic diseases (Goudge *et al.*, 2009a) sought formal care in South Africa. This study also found that among the three most frequently reported CNCDs, people with the CNCD covered by the EHP (chronic cardiovascular conditions) sought more formal care than those with CNCDs not covered by the EHP (chronic pains and chronic respiratory conditions). This suggests that the EHP might have a certain role in encouraging people to seek formal care. However, considering that more than 90% of those seeking formal care opted for public facilities where all health care is supposed to be free of charge and where the EHP is mainly delivered, the effect of free health care organized by the Malawian government in providing adequate access to CNCD care is limited.

This study also found that around 7% of those reporting CNCDs chose traditional care. The relatively low use of traditional care identified in this study is in line with a recent study on maternal care in Malawi indicating that only 2% out of 1812 women who had a pregnancy/pregnancies during the last 12 months prior to the survey date used traditional care for delivery (Mazalale *et al.*, forthcoming). Other studies from South Africa also revealed a small proportion of the population using traditional care in a setting where health care is delivered free of charge at governmental clinics (Nxumalo *et al.*, 2011; Lopes Ibanez-Gonzalez and Norris, 2013). The low use of traditional care reported in this study suggests that the free health care system in Malawi curbs peoples' demand for traditional care to a certain extent.

In addition, about 15% of those reporting CNCDs opted for home treatment. This figure seems to not be sizable compared with other studies reporting that over 35% of respondents with CNCDs bought drugs from stores as their way of treating CNCDs in other countries in SSA (Chuma *et al.*, 2007; Faronbi *et al.*, 2014). However, considering that health care in my study setting is officially free of charge at point of use and already 40% of respondents with CNCDs in my sample already chose no treatment, the use of home treatment by people with CNCDs identified in this study is still considerable.

4.3.3 Factors associated with health seeking behavior on CNCDs

Only a few selected factors were found to be significantly associated with service use, those being illness severity and duration, suffering from an "early detectable CNCD", SES, being a household head, and the proportion of household members with a CNCD living in a household.

The bivariate analysis showed that CNCDs with a detectable subclinical phase (early detectable CNCDs) were perceived to be more severe and of shorter duration compared to CNCDs without this latent phase (established CNCDs). The early detectable CNCDs group entails individuals who, at least in part, were made aware of subclinical pathology through participation in screening programs in the absence of illness symptoms. As the duration of the subclinical stage can be prolonged depending on individuals' risk factor modulation and treatment compliance, symptomatic illness occurs on average at a later stage which might explain the shorter duration of actual disease awareness in this group.

With respect to perceived illness severity, the bivariate analysis showed that on average more individuals with early detectable CNCDs considered their chronic condition hindering their routine activities compared to individuals in the established CNCD group. The finding might reflect the fact that chronic conditions diagnosed during subclinical stages, although symptom-free and thus less apparent to an individual in terms of severity, still result in early awareness, clinical enrolment, risk factor modulation and treatment compliance. Unlike individuals with chronic ailments that are not the focus of diagnostic screening programs, those with early detectable CNCDs perceive the consequences as strong limitations to their daily activities.

Taken together the findings on perceived severity, disease duration, and disease classification suggest that individuals do not necessarily seek care for chronic conditions once they are affected in their daily performance, but that the longer they live with a disease, the less likely they are to perceive this disease as problematic and therefore to act upon it. This might be of limited relevance for chronic complaints that have little or no direct link to premature mortality (e.g. chronic muscle or joint pain, chronic skin disorders, chronic digestive problems, chronic respiratory diseases, chronic psychiatric or psycho-somatic disorders) and/or are widely accepted as age-related ailments (e.g. loss of vision, loss of hearing, senile dementia, etc.). This finding, however, is worrisome in a context of chronic conditions due to cardiovascular, metabolic, or common neoplastic processes, as epidemiological studies have suggested being the case in Malawi (Msyamboza et al., 2011, 2012). The fact that early detectable CNCDs are more severe but with shorter duration than other CNCDs suggests that people with these diseases in Malawi do not obtain proper screening and treatment services and had more financial burden although the services of these diseases should be freely provided by the EHP. For such conditions, non-compliance after early detection of risk factors or mild disease states can easily contribute to rapid progression with important effects on premature disability and mortality at younger age (World Health Organization, 2011a). Given the high levels of seeking no care among chronically ill individuals, further research is needed on the perceptions of Malawians about CNCDs in order to develop patient-centered screen-and-treat strategies within existing health service programs (van der Sande et al., 2001; Lim et al., 2007).

Given the paucity of studies on factors associated with health seeking for CNCDs from other SSA settings, it is of value to enlarge the scope of discussion from CNCDs to acute conditions. In line with prior studies on treatment seeking behavior on CNCDs from Tanzania, Uganda, and South Africa (Kidanto et al., 2002; Kazaura et al., 2007; Goudge et al., 2009a; Petricca et al., 2009; Hjelm and Atwine, 2011; Osamor, 2011; Birhanu et al., 2012), this study revealed that perceived severity was both significantly associated with an increased likelihood of utilizing formal and informal care. Not surprisingly, this suggests that perceived severity is as important an element in influencing health seeking decisions for chronic conditions in the region as it has long been recognized to be for acute conditions (MacKian, 2003; Gotsadze et al., 2005; Dong et al., 2008).

Interestingly, respondents with longer duration of CNCDs were found to seek less formal care than those with shorter duration. Duration of disease did not influence the utilization of informal care. These results suggest that people with longer duration of CNCDs in Malawi have poor continuity of care for CNCDs, which aligns with evidence related to the role of duration of disease on treating and controlling CNCDs in LMICs (Gimenes et al., 2009; Khattab et al., 2010; Mukherjee et al., 2011; Ramli et al., 2012). Considering that longer duration of CNCDs is usually linked with higher severity of the disease and people with longer duration of CNCDs usually know more about how to control and treat these conditions (Norfazilah et al., 2013), the negative effect of duration of disease on utilization of formal care is really quite alarming, especially in an officially free health care system.

My original hypothesis postulated expected that individuals suffering from early detectable CNCDs would be more likely to seek formal care, given that screening and risk factor modulation programs are in principle available within the EHP. The analysis, however, did not detect such an effect, but only identified a preference among these individuals towards not seeking informal care (when compared to no care). This finding from MNL model coincided with the result of bivariate analysis of perceived severity, disease duration, and disease classification in this dissertation. Both results from bivariate analysis and MNL model suggest that under the EHP, which is designed to improve access of care in an officially free health care system in Malawi, access to services related to CNCDs remains erratic. In controlling premature mortality resulting from chronic diseases, especially such CNCDs preventable or modifiable by early detection and targeted drug therapy, patient compliance with provider follow-up and medical regimens is paramount. In settings where health resource limitations and access barriers might jeopardize this continuity of chronic care, acceleration of disease progression in early life is a commonly observed outcome (World Health Organization, 2005, 2011a).

SES was found to be associated with both the decision to seek informal care and the decision to seek formal care. The size of the coefficients, however, indicated that SES had relative little weight compared to other factors. The relative little weight of SES in shaping care decisions appeared surprising since it overtly contradicts the large body of evidence on health seeking in SSA for both chronic (Alberts et al., 2003) and acute conditions (Fosu, 1994; Chuma et al., 2007; Dong et al., 2008; Kolling et al., 2010), as it suggested smaller inequities in access due to SES than in most other SSA countries. The secondary importance of SES in comparison to other settings can most likely be explained in relation to existing health system structures, providing care "free of charge", at least in principle. Appraising jointly the effect of SES and of disease classification, described just above, seems to suggest that system barriers to access do exist, but are probably not the financial resources that a household owns. They are possibly more related to the actual availability and quality of services included in the EHP. This requires further qualitative research, approaching the issue from a supply rather than demand perspective.

On the one hand, being a household head was also found to be positively associated with seeking either formal or informal care. This finding was by no means surprising since it aligns with a literature on SSA, indicating that intra-household allocation of resources for health prioritizes productive household members (Sauerborn et al., 1996), specifically the family head (Su et al., 2006b; Dong et al., 2008). On the other hand, living in a household with a higher proportion of household members suffering from a CNCD was negatively associated with seeking either formal or informal care. This finding was also not surprising. It indicated that intra-household resource allocation is obviously more problematic when multiple family members suffer from conditions which rely on continuity of care and which may therefore result in sustained high spending.

4.3.4 OOP expenditure on CNCDs

In line with prior studies (Zere et al., 2010; Mwandira, 2011), my findings confirmed that about two-thirds of people suffering from a CNCD still incurred OOP expenditure on direct medical and travel costs, in spite of a system which, in principle, should offer essential care free of charge at point of use. This study also demonstrated that among the three most frequently reported CNCDs, OOP expenditure on the CNCD covered by the EHP (chronic cardiovascular conditions), which is prioritized to be delivered free of charge in Malawi, was much higher than that on CNCDs not covered by the EHP (chronic pains and chronic respiratory conditions). In addition, spending on direct medical and travel costs were found to account for a considerable proportion of monthly per capita household spending, which is consistent with studies on overall OOP expenditure on CNCDs in SSA (Elrayah et al., 2005; Chuma et al., 2007; Obi and Ozumba, 2008; Goudge et al., 2009a; Elrayah-Eliadarous et al., 2010; Huffman et al., 2011). These findings indicate that choosing to treat a chronic condition in Malawi still imposes an important financial burden on rural poor households. For many other households (nearly 40% in the sample), the cost of seeking care might have been the reason deterring utilization in the first place (Haque et al., 2005; World Health Organization, 2005; Goudge et al., 2009a). Interestingly, prior research showed that the drug prices for chronic conditions in Malawi are substantially higher than in most other LMICs (Mendis et al.,

2007). This appears paradoxical given the existence of a system that is supposed to provide basic healthcare services, including medications, free of charge.

This study also showed that more than 60% of those who incurred OOP expenditure did not spend anything on transportation, suggesting that direct medical expenditure, but not travel cost, is the main source for the high OOP expenditure for CNCDs in the study area. This is similar to the results indicating that travel cost accounts for less than 5% of the total direct cost for diabetes in Tanzania (Chale *et al.*, 1992) and for chronic obstructive pulmonary disease and hypertension in Bangladesh (Uddin *et al.*, 2014). This finding, however, is contradictory with other studies indicating that OOP expenditure is mostly related to transportation cost for acute diseases in Malawi (Kemp *et al.*, 2007) and for general conditions or maternal care in a free or user-fee exempted system in SSA (Kruk *et al.*, 2008; Goudge *et al.*, 2009b). The less prominent role of travel cost on overall OOP expenditure can be explained by the fact that drugs for treating CNCDs are extremely expensive on a continuous basis of use and account for the largest share of the total direct cost, which is frequently reported by studies on OOP expenditure for CNCDs in SSA (Chale *et al.*, 1992; Elrayah *et al.*, 2005; Odili and Okwuanasor, 2012) and in LMICs (Kankeu *et al.*, 2013).

This study further found that although travel cost was not the driving force for the total OOP expenditure for CNCD, it was the only source of cost that differentiated the total OOP expenditure between the two care options with clients incurring much lower transport costs for informal care than formal care. Somewhat surprising is the fact that OOP expenditure on direct medical costs did not differ substantially between individuals using formal and informal care. This may be explained in relation to the fact that people visiting facilities may still be asked to purchase drugs OOP exactly as those individuals choosing directly self-treatment, purchasing medications at private pharmacies. Drug shortages at public facilities have already been reported to be frequent in the Malawian context (Mueller et al. 2011; National Statistical Office Malawi 2011) and to be one of the major drivers of household OOP spending on health in SSA (Mugisha *et al.*, 2002). Prior evidence would appear to support this hypothesis since it indicated that in 2005, only 5% of drugs needed to treat common chronic conditions were available at public Malawian health facilities (Mendis *et al.*, 2007).

Appraising findings on direct medical costs and findings on travel costs together suggest that some households may opt for self-treatment in the first place knowing that travelling to a facility bears a high risk of resulting in a higher overall OOP expenditure, if the facility is not equipped as it should to provide services free of charge within the framework of the EHP.

Another important finding in this study related to OOP expenditure on CNCD is that the poorer quartile spent a considerably higher proportion of their monthly per capita household expenditure on healthcare needs related to CNCDs than wealthier quartiles. This finding is consistent with prior studies in Malawi (Kemp *et al.*, 2007; Mwandira, 2011) and in other LMICs (Su *et al.*, 2006b; Kankeu *et al.*, 2013; Rahman *et al.*, 2013), indicating that OOP expenditure on healthcare is generally regressive. This finding is particularly worrisome since the negative effect of regressive payments for health has been widely documented in the literature (Xu *et al.*, 2003; Gottret and Schieber, 2006).

In addition, my findings also revealed that a considerable proportion of households incurred catastrophic spending due to CNCDs. The poorest households faced the highest risk of catastrophic spending due to CNCDs. This finding, which relies on OOP expenditure for CNCDs aggregated at the household level, support findings from the descriptive analysis related to OOP expenditure shown above, which pointed at the regressivity of individual out-of-pocket expenditure on CNCDs. This finding is also consistent with prior analyses of catastrophic spending, which included chronic conditions as an explanatory variable in models targeting the overall economic burden due to ill health in SSA (Su *et al.*, 2006a; Xu *et al.*, 2006b) and in LMICs more in general (Engelgau *et al.*, 2012; Jiang *et al.*, 2012; Rahman *et al.*, 2013; Gotsadze *et al.*, 2009; Van Minh and Xuan Tran, 2012). These studies had already indicated how suffering from a chronic condition represented an important determinant of catastrophic spending.

Meanwhile, this study found that an additional 1.7% of households with at least one household member reporting a CNCD fell under the international poverty line once expenditures due to CNCDs were considered. The fact that the economic burden of CNCDs aggravates poverty is in line with previous studies focusing specifically on the economic impact of CNCDs on affected households (Bhojani *et al.*, 2012; Le *et al.*, 2012) and using CNCDs as an explanatory variable influencing the incidence of impoverishment

(Xu *et al.*, 2006b; Engelgau *et al.*, 2012; Jiang *et al.*, 2012; Van Minh and Xuan Tran, 2012) in LMICs. In the context of Malawi, this finding appears worrisome in light of the rapid growth of CNCDs and the fact that above 40% of households already live below the international poverty line.

4.3.5 Factors associated with OOP expenditure on CNCDs

The two-part model allowed this study to identify various factors that shape an individual's risk of incurring higher OOP expenditure when chronically ill. Those determinants show similarities as well as differences with the determinants found to drive OOP expenditure on non-chronic conditions (Su *et al.*, 2006b; Okunade *et al.*, 2010; Onwujekwe *et al.*, 2010; Malik and Syed, 2012; Rahman *et al.*, 2013; Yardim *et al.*, 2014).

In line with prior studies (Su *et al.*, 2006b; Malik and Syed, 2012; Schwarz *et al.*, 2013; Yardim *et al.*, 2014), the findings in this dissertation revealed that the wealthier the household, the higher the OOP expenditure on CNCDs. In the dissertation, however, the role played by SES in shaping OOP expenditure on CNCDs was less prominent than usually found in the literature. Similarly, as shown previously, the role of SES in this Malawian setting was also less prominent in influencing health seeking behavior for CNCDs, which might indicate that SES in this context might be less important in explaining the differences in OOP expenditure on CNCDs. In a system which, at least in principle, provides care free of charge at point of use, absolute differences in OOP expenditure across SES quartiles are likely to be lower than in systems that structurally rely on user fee charges. Meanwhile, also in line with prior empirical analyses on household health expenditure (Getzen, 2000; Okunade *et al.*, 2010), the income elasticity, estimated based on the SES coefficient in the two-part model, was inelastic or near to zero. This implies that a 1% rise in income will lead to far less than a 1% increase in OOP expenditure, also indicating the less prominent role of SES in directly shaping OOP expenditure on CNCDs in Malawi.

In the analysis, use of formal care was positively associated with both the probability of incurring and the magnitude of incurred OOP expenditure on CNCDs. This indicates that the overall level of OOP spending was higher among users of formal than among users of informal care. Again, in a context where essential care is supposedly provided free of charge at point of use, and where the vast majority of those using formal services actually use public facilities (more than 90% in the sample of this dissertation), this finding indicates important gaps in service coverage and financial protection as recently identified by a parallel qualitative study (Abiiro et al., 2014). In principle, those who choose to use public facilities should be able to access essential care, including laboratory tests and drugs, free of charge and should be left to pay only for transportation costs. This dissertation already found the higher OOP expenditure among users of formal care is driven by direct medical expenditure, suggesting that tests and drugs are not always available free of charge, probably due to underfunding at the system level (Ministry of Health Malawi, 2011). Further qualitative investigation is necessary to understand if higher OOP spending is incurred because patients are charged informal fees or because they are sent to private structures to purchase material which is missing at public facilities. In either case, the expectation of ultimately facing higher costs if seeking formal rather than informal care may very well act as a deterrent when making decisions on how to treat CNCDs (Kankeu et al., 2013), potentially leading to improper disease management and worse long-term health outcomes (World Health Organization, 2005).

The analysis on health seeking behavior for CNCDs indicated that people with CNCDs targeted by EHP free screening programs did not seek more formal care, but sought less informal care than those with CNCDs not targeted by such programs. The analysis on expenditure confirmed that suffering from CNCDs targeted by EHP screening programs was negatively associated with the possibility of incurring OOP expenditure but positively associated with the magnitude of OOP expenditure. This finding appeared surprising, since this study expected to observe a lower level OOP expenditure on CNCDs targeted by the EHP, due to the fact that an explicit aim of the EHP is to serve as a financial protection mechanism against illness-induced costs. The opposite findings suggest that the EHP, as currently implemented, has very limited effects on removing the financial burden induced by selected CNCDs. A possible explanation for this surprising finding may be found by looking at the literature, which has amply documented a general inability of the system to provide services in the quantity and quality stipulated by the EHP (Bowie and Mwase, 2011; Mueller et al., 2011).

Contradicting prior evidence on acute conditions (Su *et al.*, 2006b; Orem *et al.*, 2013), this dissertation found perceived disease severity to be positively associated with the probability of incurring OOP expenditure, but not with the magnitude of the expenditure. In line with prior studies (Shobhana *et al.*, 2000; Ramachandran *et al.*, 2007; Trogdon and Hylands, 2008), illness duration was instead found to be positively associated with the magnitude of OOP expenditure. These findings indicate that perceived illness severity, although relevant for an individual's perceived quality of life, is less suitable for representing actual severity of disease than illness duration for the purpose of analyzing OOP expenditure on CNCDs. The fact that illness duration is an important predictor of OOP expenditure on CNCDs is not surprising, since CNCDs normally aggravate with time and thus require more intense medical care (World Health Organization, 2005). From the standpoint of financial protection, this obviously calls into question the capacity of the Malawian healthcare system to cater for individuals who need relatively expensive lifelong care, while still struggling to curb mortality due to infectious diseases and lack of qualified maternal care (National Statistical Office (Malawi), 2011).

The positive association detected between being a household head and the amount of OOP spending on CNCDs aligns with the vast body of evidence indicating that the intra-household allocation of resources for health in SSA prioritizes productive household members (Sauerborn *et al.*, 1996) and particularly the family head (Su *et al.*, 2006b; Onwujekwe *et al.*, 2010). Given that this study controlled for age, it is unlikely that the effect detected reflects individual CNCD risk profiles, but more likely that it reflects actual preferences on intra-household resource allocation. Similarly, consistent both with theoretical models of demand for health care (Grossman, 1972) and with prior empirical studies from LMICs (Su *et al.*, 2006b; Okunade *et al.*, 2010; Malik and Syed, 2012; Rahman *et al.*, 2013; Yardim *et al.*, 2014), this study found that OOP expenditure was higher among individuals whose household head was literate. Literate household heads have better access to health information. This is likely to result in better health knowledge and, in turn, in different decisions regarding investments in health. Living in a household with a higher proportion of individuals suffering from a chronic illness was negatively associated with the magnitude of individual OOP expenditure on CNCDs. This finding is not surprising.

Households with multiple family members suffering from one or more CNCDs usually have fewer resources for each affected household member, given that in a context of generalized poverty, limited resources have to be shared between many individuals.

In line with previous studies analyzing OOP expenditure for general conditions in Tanzania (Brinda *et al.*, 2014) and for chronic obstructive pulmonary disease and hypertension in Bangladesh (Uddin *et al.*, 2014), being female was found to be positively associated with the level of OOP expenditure for CNCDs after controlling for other factors. As to how to explain the role of gender on OOP expenditure on CNCDs, the study from Tanzania attributed the positive correlates of OOP expenditure and being female to women's needs on reproductive health care (Brinda *et al.*, 2014), which is not the case for this study since it has narrowed down to the analysis of OOP expenditure on CNCDs only, i.e. the outcome variable in the analysis excluded the cost on reproductive care. The second study from Bangladesh found that due to the fact that women used more care provided by trained health staff, women incurred higher OOP expenditure for chronic obstructive pulmonary disease and hypertension than men (Uddin *et al.*, 2014). This explanation, however, is not applicable to this study since women in my sample were not found to use more formal or informal care for CNCDs than men. Further qualitative inquiry is needed to deeply understand why women in my study setting incurred higher OOP expenditure on CNCDs than men.

In addition, being Alomwe was also found to be positively associated with the amount of OOP expenditure on CNCDs. As the dominant ethnic group in the study area, it is possible that the Alomwe are more frequently and intensively exposed to health promotion programs, thus being more aware of their health needs and being more willing to spend more once they come into contact with the healthcare system. Further qualitative inquiry is also needed to thoroughly understand the role of ethnicity in health spending on CNCDs and thus draft adequate policy recommendations.

4.4 Generalizability of research findings

Two major methods are available to provide evidence for generalizability: the sampling model and proximal similarity model. The former refers to generalizing the results to the source population by drawing a representative sample from the population. The latter refers to generalizing the findings beyond the source population whose setting is more or less similar to that of the source population. Proximal similarity model is often used in social science since social scientists are more interested in generalizing the experience from the study area to other settings (Campbell, 1986; Phillips *et al.*, 2013). As an explorative study exploring health seeking behavior and OOP expenditure on CNCDs in SSA, it makes more sense that my thesis uses the proximal similarity model to discuss generalizability. By providing every detail related to the study context, other researchers could fully understand similarities and differences between my study setting and the specific context that they concern and make decisions on whether my findings can be generalized to their context.

Similar to other districts in Malawi, in my study area, Thyolo, Chiradzulu, and Mulanje districts, health care is provided free of charge at point of use, which is different from most settings in SSA. Therefore, one needs to be especially cautious when generalizing the results from this study to a context that mainly relies on user fees. However, my study setting is not unlike many other rural areas in SSA. First, the majority of the continent in SSA is generally poor and relies on subsistence agriculture which also represents the main economic activity in the study area. Second, similar to my study area, the disease burden due to CNCDs is increasing in SSA (Aït-Khaled *et al.*, 2001; Tsang *et al.*, 2008; Msyamboza *et al.*, 2009; de Ramirez *et al.*, 2010; Miszkurka *et al.*, 2012), leaving countries in the region facing a double burden of disease (Unwin *et al.*, 2001; Boutayeb and Boutayeb, 2005; Dalal *et al.*, 2011). Third, considering the generally limited capacity of health provision systems and poor financial protection from CNCD-induced cost in the region (World Health Organization Regional Office for Africa, 2011), one can conclude that people in most countries in SSA face similar barriers to care related to CNCDs and have to bear a high financial burden due to these diseases through OOP payment, as confirmed in this study even within a setting where health care is provided free of charge at point of use. Fourth, I trust that the household head plays a decisive role in allocating resources within households in most settings in SSA as indicated in my analysis (Sauerborn *et al.*, 1996; Su *et al.*, 2006b; Dong *et al.*, 2008; Onwujekwe *et al.*, 2010).

4.5 Policy implications and recommendations

The overall goal of this dissertation was to provide systematic evidence on patterns and determinants of health seeking behavior and OOP expenditure for CNCDs in SSA, which constitutes an important basis for policy formulation and intervention development for CNCDs in the region.

This study found that a large proportion of people with CNCDs in rural Malawi did not use any care, people with CNCDs were more likely to seek care when they felt their conditions to be severe, and people with CNCDs targeted by the EHP did not seek more formal care. On the one hand, these findings related to health seeking behavior indicate that including the most common CNCDs into the EHP, the only intervention that Malawi has taken for CNCDs till now, is not sufficient to ensure adequate provision of care. First, the Malawian government needs to find out the reasons explaining the gap between the policy and the reality and then make a policy adjustment in order to provide better services related to CNCDs. On the other hand, considering that no specific intervention for CNCDs is available in Malawi till now, this study suggests that the Malawian government needs to develop more integrated interventions specifically targeting CNCDs, yet feasible within the existing health system. Taking the nature of chronic diseases into consideration, the core element for care related to chronic diseases is to change the progression of disease by training people to become activated agents for the best of their own health (Coleman *et al.*, 2009). A comprehensive set of interventions are developed by Westerns countries to help people become actively and informed towards CNCDs. These interventions, either population-based or individual-based, range from the nonmedical sector such as laws, regulations, tax, price, and advocacy, to medical sectors involving activities such as screening, clinical prevention, habilitation and so on (World Health Organization, 2005). The WHO has already recommended several 'best buy' interventions that are suitable in resource-restricted countries with an annual per capita cost of under US$ 1 in low-income settings and between US$ 1.50 to US$ 3 in middle-income countries (World Health Organization, 2011d). All these recommended interventions by the WHO need not be implemented immediately in these settings. A stepwise implementation ought to be adopted based on local priorities and contexts in the region. Apart from the WHO recommended interventions for resource-limited countries, much attention should be paid to other localized successful lessons related to treatment and control for CNCDs in the region; such as, to train traditional healers to identify suspected cases for CNCDs and to refer them early to formal care since traditional care is widely applied in SSA (Mbeh *et al.*, 2010). As well they should train general duty nurses in the rural areas to provide care at the patients' home with regular support from hospital doctors (Mamo *et al.*, 2007).

In light of the findings indicating a substantial financial burden imposed by CNCDs to the local population in an officially free health care system, this study indicates that in a resource-limited country like Malawi only relying on state-funded financing cannot provide adequate financial protection against the cost on CNCDs. Complementary health insurance, though underdeveloped now in Malawi, is expected to play an important role in risk pooling for CNCDs (Makoka *et al.*, 2007; Phiri and Masanjala, 2012). Learning from other LMICs where the government's capability to establish and run a state-funded financing and social health insurance system is restrained by its social-economic development (Preker *et al.*, 2004). Micro health insurance (MHI) has proved to reduce OOP expenditure as well as increase access to care (Criel and Dormael, 1999; Dror and Jacquier, 1999; Carrin, 2003), especially in the rural areas in LMICs (Adebayo *et al.*, 2014). In the rural setting in Malawi, MHI schemes are encouraged to be developed (Makoka *et al.*, 2007). Considering that the literature has frequently reported a strong causal relationship between CNCDs and poverty (World Health Organization, 2005; Su *et al.*, 2006a; Gotsadze *et al.*, 2009; Sun *et al.*, 2009; Engelgau *et al.*, 2012; Van Minh and Xuan Tran, 2012; Kankeu *et al.*, 2013; Rahman *et al.*, 2013; Xu *et al.*, 2006b) and no MHI in SSA, to our knowledge, covers the cost CNCDs, this study suggests the local policy makers to include CNCDs in the benefit package of MHI. Based on the findings from this study, the benefit package of MHI regarding CNCDs should prioritize the services leading to direct medical costs, but not the travel cost. This study also clearly revealed that the poorest people run the highest risk of becoming impoverished due to CNCDs in an officially free health system. Looking outside Malawi, it is often reported that the poor are still under worse financial protection against illness-induced cost than the wealthy in a setting where only the poor are exempted from any user fees (Ridde *et al.*, 2014) or where all of the population is entitled to the removal of user fees

(Xu *et al.*, 2006a). In line with policy suggestions proposed by a study on the household financial burden on tuberculosis in Malawi (Kemp *et al.*, 2007), this study suggests that to better financially protect the poor against CNCD-induced cost it is necessary to go beyond providing free health care for the poor or removing their user fees, but instead renovating the way that care for CNCDs are delivered for the poor. Future investigation, both from the government and the academic society, is needed to develop innovative interventions to deliver CNCD care for the poor.

It took HICs more than a century to adapt the transitions due to the growing burden of CNCDs. However, these transitions are taking place very quickly in LMICs, especially in SSA, leaving insufficient time for them to adapt (Kengne *et al.*, 2013). In SSA, to cope with the burden of CNCDs is even more complex since the burden of acute communicable diseases is still very heavy (Unwin *et al.*, 2001; Boutayeb and Boutayeb, 2005; Dalal *et al.*, 2011). Policy makers in the region ought to first understand the current situation of CNCDs and the need of the population, and then formulate evidence-based interventions to prevent and control CNCDs (Mendis, 2010; Chan *et al.*, 2012). This explorative study describes the status quo of health seeking behavior and OOP expenditure on CNCDs in Malawi, which can be used as the basic information for developing interventions for CNCDs in the setting. However, further studies are needed to help the country to draft policies and fight against CNCDs.

5. Conclusions

This study indicated that CNCDs impose a considerable burden on households in Malawi. In spite of a 'free' health care system, only one third of all respondents affected by a CNCD sought formal care. Seeking care, whether formal or informal, was associated with high OOP expenditure on both medical and travel costs. The financial burden of CNCDs leads households to face catastrophic spending and pushes households further into poverty. The poor population bore the highest financial burden caused by CNCDs. Though screening and treatment for several CNCDs are in principle covered by the EHP, the low utilization rates and the high financial burden due to CNCDs detected in the study suggest the existence of important gaps in service coverage and financial protection in the current government's universal health coverage policy. Existing policy needs to translate into direct action plans to ensure that in a context of generalized poverty, households facing multiple health burdens (from acute, chronic, and maternal conditions) benefit from proper access to the services and adequate financial protection. Further qualitative research is needed to thoroughly understand the reasons motivating low service utilization and high financial burden imposed by CNCDs in a basically free health system and to explore probably supply-side barriers to access.

6. Summary

CNCDs already present a considerable burden in SSA. Health system in SSA struggle to cope with service provision and financial protection related to CNCDs. In order to respond to this rising 'epidemic', more research on CNCDs are needed to help health systems in SSA to be restructured.

This study was based in rural Malawi and designed to address two sets of questions:

1) What are the patterns of health seeking behavior on CNCDs in rural Malawi? Which factors are associated with treatment options for these conditions?
2) What are the patterns of OOP expenditure on CNCDs in rural Malawi? Which factors are associated with OOP expenditure on these conditions? What is the economic impact of OOP expenditure on CNCDs?

In order to answer the above questions, I analyzed data from the first round of a panel household health survey on a total sample of 1199 households between August and October 2012 in the rural districts of Thyolo, Chiradzulu, and Mulanje. I used descriptive statistics to describe treatment options and related household OOP expenditure on CNCDs. I carried out MNL and a two-part model to analyze factors associated with health seeking behavior and OOP expenditure on CNCDs.

This study found that a total of 475 respondents reported at least one CNCD. Among them, 37.3% did not seek any care, 42.5% sought formal care, and 20.2% opted for informal care. Regression analysis showed that illness severity and duration, SES, being a household head, and the proportion of household members living with a CNCD were significantly associated with health care utilization.

Out of 475 respondents reporting CNCDs, more than 40% incurred OOP expenditure. The amount of OOP expenditure on CNCDs comprised 22% of their monthly per capita household expenditure. The poorer the household, the higher proportion of their monthly per capita household expenditure was spent on CNCDs. Using a threshold of 10% of household non-food expenditure, 21.3% of all households with at least one household member reporting a CNCD and seeking care for such a condition incurred catastrophic spending due to CNCDs. An additional 1.7% of households reporting a CNCD fell under the international poverty line once considering the direct costs due to CNCDs. Higher severity of disease and use of formal care were significantly associated with an increased likelihood of incurring OOP expenditure. Suffering from a CNCD targeted by EHP screening was negatively associated with the possibility of incurring OOP expenditure. The following factors were positively associated with the amount of OOP expenditure: being female, Alomwe and a household head, longer duration of disease, CNCDs targeted through active screening programs, higher SES, household head being literate, using formal care, and fewer household members living with a CNCD within a household.

This study is important as it is one of the first studies exploring determinants of health seeking behavior and OOP expenditure on CNCDs in SSA. My findings showed that, in spite of a context where care for CNCDs should in principle be available free of charge at point of use, the utilization rates of care related to CNCCs are still low and OOP payments impose a considerable financial burden on rural households, especially among the poorest. To increase access to care and provide financial protection for people suffering from CNCDs, the provision of a free Essential Health Package in Malawi ought to be strengthened through the integration of system-wide screening, risk factor modification, and continuity of care options for people suffering from CNCDs.

7. References

Abegunde DO, Stanciole AE. 2008. The Economic Impact of Chronic Diseases. How do Households Respond to Shocks? Evidence From Russia. *Social Science and Medicine* **66**: 2296–307.

Abiiro GA, Mbera GB, De Allegri M. 2014. Gaps in Universal Health Coverage in Malawi. A Qualitative Study in Rural Communities. *BMC Health Services Research* **14**.

Acock AC. 2008. Multiple regression. In: *A Gentle Introduction to Stata, third edition.* Stata Press: College Station, Texas, 243–88.

Addo J, Agyemang C, Smeeth L, de-Graft Aikins A, Edusei AK, Ogedegbe O. 2012. A review of population-based studies on hypertension in Ghana. *Ghana Medical Journal* **46**: 4–11.

Adebayo EF, Ataguba JE, Uthman OA, Okwundu CI, Lamont KT, Wiysonge CS. 2014. Factors that affect the uptake of community-based health insurance in low-income and middle-income countries: a systematic protocol. *BMJ Open* **4**: e004167.

Africa Health Workforce Observatory. 2009. Human Resources for Health Country Profile – Malawi. World Health Organization/ Regional Office for Africa.

Aikins AG. 2007. Ghana's neglected chronic disease epidemic: a developmental challenge. *Ghana Medical Journal* **41**: 154–9.

Aït-Khaled N, Enarson D, Bousquet J. 2001. Chronic respiratory diseases in developing countries: the burden and strategies for prevention and management. *Bulletin of the World Health Organization* **79**: 971–9.

Akin JS, Guilkey DK, Denton EH. 1995. Quality of services and demand for health care in Nigeria: a multinomial probit estimation. *Social Science & Medicine* **40**: 1527–37.

Akweongo P, Dalaba MA, Hayden MH, *et al.* 2013. The Economic Burden of Meningitis to Households in Kassena-Nankana District of Northern Ghana. *PLoS ONE* **8**: e79880.

Alberts M, Olwagen R, Molaba C, Choma S. 2003. Socio-economic Status and the Diagnosis, Treatment and Control of Hypertension in the Dikgale Field Site, South Africa

Amal N, Paramesarvathy R, Tee G. 2011. Prevalence of Chronic Illness and Health Seeking Behaviour in Malaysian Population: Results from the Third National Health Morbidity Survey (NHMS III) 2006. *Medical Journal of Malaysia* **66**: 36–41.

Aspray TJ, Mugusi F, Rashid S, *et al.* 2000. Rural and Urban Differences in Diabetes Prevalence in Tanzania. The Role of Obesity, Physical Inactivity and Urban Living. *Transactions of the Royal Society of Tropical Medicine and Hygiene* **94**: 637–44.

Atif M, Sulaiman SAS, Shafie AA, Asif M, Babar Z-U-D. 2014. Resource utilization pattern and cost of tuberculosis treatment from the provider and patient perspectives in the state of Penang, Malaysia. *BMC Health Services Research* **14**: 353.

Azevedo M, Alla S. 2008. Diabetes in Sub-Saharan Africa: Kenya, Mali, Mozambique, Nigeria, South Africa and Zambia. *International Journal of Diabetes in Developing Countries* **28**: 101–8.

Baliga SS, Gopakumaran PS, Katti SM, Mallapur MD. 2013. Treatment Seeking Behavior and Health Care Expenditure Incurred for Hypertension among elderly in Urban Slums of Belgaum City. *National Journal of Community Medicine* **4**: 227–30.

Basu A, Manning WG. 2009. Issues for the next generation of health care cost analyses. *Medical care* **47**: S109–14.

Basu A, Rathouz PJ. 2005. Estimating marginal and incremental effects on health outcomes using flexible link and variance function models. *Biostatistics (Oxford, England)* **6**: 93–109.

Baum CF. 2006. *An Introduction to Modern Econometrics Using Stata.* Stata Press: College Station, Tex.

Belotti F, Deb P, Manning WG, Norton EC. 2012. tpm: Estimating Two-part Models. *The Stata Journal* **vv**: 1–13.

Beran D, Yudkin JS. 2006. Diabetes care in sub-Saharan Africa. *The Lancet* **368**: 1689–95.

Bhojani U, Beerenahalli TS, Devadasan R, *et al.* 2013. No longer diseases of the wealthy: prevalence and health-seeking for self-reported chronic conditions among urban poor in Southern India. *BMC Health Services Research* **13**: 306.

Bhojani U, Bs T, Devadasan R, *et al.* 2012. Out-of-Pocket Healthcare Payments on Chronic Conditions Impoverish Urban Poor in Bangalore, India. *BMC Public Health* **12**: 990.

Birhanu Z, Abdissa A, Belachew T, *et al.* 2012. Health seeking behavior for cervical cancer in Ethiopia: a qualitative study. *International Journal for Equity in Health* **11**: 1–8.

Bloom D, Cafiero E, Jané-Llopis E. 2011. The Global Economic Burden of Non-communicable Diseases. Harvard School of Public Health, Cambridge, MA.

Bolduc D, Lacroix G, Muller C. 1996. The choice of medical providers in rural Bénin: a comparison of discrete choice models. *Journal of Health Economics* **15**: 477–98.

Borah BJ. 2006. A mixed logit model of health care provider choice: analysis of NSS data for rural India. *Health Economics* **15**: 915–32.

Boutayeb A, Boutayeb S. 2005. The burden of non-communicable diseases in developing countries. *International Journal for Equity in Health* **4**: 2.

Bowie C, Mwase T. 2011. Assessing the Use of an Essential Health Package in a Sector Wide Approach in Malawi. *Health Research Policy and Systems* **9**: 1–10.

Bowie C, Richardson A, Sykes W. 1995. Consulting the Public About Health Service Priorities. *British Medical Journal* **311**: 1155–8.

Box GEP, Cox DR. 1964. An Analysis of Transformations. *Journal of the Royal Statistical Society. Series B (Methodological)* **26**: 211–52.

Bradshaw D, Norman R, Pieterse D, Levitt NS, Collaboration SACRA. 2007. Estimating the burden of disease attributable to diabetes in South Africa in 2000. *South African Medical Journal* **97**: 700–706.

Brinda E, Andrés R, Enemark U. 2014. Correlates of out-of-pocket and catastrophic health expenditures in Tanzania: results from a national household survey. *BMC International Health and Human Rights* **14**: 5.

Brown PH, Theoharides C. 2009. Health-seeking behavior and hospital choice in China's New Cooperative Medical System. *Health Economics* **18**: S47–S64.

Cameron AC, Trivedi PK. 2005. *Microeconometrics. Methods and Applications.* Cambridge University Press: Cambridge, New York u.a.

Cameron AC, Trivedi PK. 2010. *Microeconometrics Using Stata*. Stata Press: College Station, Tex.

Campbell DT. 1986. Relabeling internal and external validity for applied social scientists. *New Directions for Program Evaluation* **1986**: 67–77.

Carrin G. 2003. Community Based Health Insurance Schemes in Developing Countries. Facts, Problems and Perspectives. Discussion Paper No. 1. World Health Organization (WHO), Geneva, Switzerland.

Cavanagh P, Attinger C, Abbas Z, Bal A, Rojas N, Xu Z-R. 2012. Cost of treating diabetic foot ulcers in five different countries. *Diabetes/Metabolism Research and Reviews* **28**: 107–11.

Central Intelligence Agency (USA). 2014. The World Factbook, Malawi.

Chadza E. 2012. Factors that contribute to delay in seeking cervical cancer diagnosis and treatment among women in Malawi. *Health* **4**: 1015–22.

Chale SS, Swai AB, Mujinja PG, McLarty DG. 1992. Must diabetes be a fatal disease in Africa? Study of costs of treatment. *BMJ (Clinical research ed.)* **304**: 1215–8.

Chan KY, Adeloye D, Grant L, Kolcic I, Marusic A. 2012. How big is the 'next big thing'? Estimating the burden of non-communicable diseases in low- and middle-income countries. *Journal of Global Health* **2**: 20101.

Chibwana AI, Mathanga DP, Chinkhumba J, Campbell CH. 2009. Socio-Cultural Predictors of Health-Seeking Behaviour for Febrile Under-Five Children in Mwanza-Neno District, Malawi. *Malaria Journal* **8**: 219–27.

Chirwa ML, Kazanga I, Faedo G, Thomas S. 2013. Promoting universal financial protection: contracting faith-based health facilities to expand access – lessons learned from Malawi. *Health Research Policy and Systems* **11**: 27.

Christiadi, Cushing BJ. 2007. Conditional Logit, IIA, and Alternatives for Estimating Models of Interstate Migration. Working Paper No. 200704. Regional Research Institute, West Virginia University.

Chuma J, Maina T. 2012. Catastrophic Health Care Spending and Impoverishment in Kenya. *BMC Health Services Research* **12**: 413.

Chuma J, Gilson L, Molyneux C. 2007. Treatment-Seeking Behaviour, Cost Burdens and Coping Strategies Among Rural and Urban Households in Coastal Kenya: an Equity Analysis. *Tropical Medicine and International Health* **12**: 673–86.

130

Cohen S, Carlson B. 1994. A Comparison of Household and Medical Provider Reported Expenditures in the 1987 NMES. *Journal of Official Statistics* **10**: 3–29.

Coleman K, Austin BT, Brach C, Wagner EH. 2009. Evidence on the Chronic Care Model in the new millennium. *Health Affairs* **28**: 75–85.

Cooper RS, Rotimi CN, Kaufman JS, Muna WF, Mensah GA. 1998. Hypertension treatment and control in sub-Saharan Africa: the epidemiological basis for policy. *BMJ : British Medical Journal* **316**: 614–7.

Criel B, Dormael M. 1999. Mutual Health Organizations in Africa and Social Health Insurance Systems. Will European History Repeat Itself? *Tropical Medicine and International Health* **4**: 155–9.

Daar AS, Singer PA, Persad DL, *et al.* 2007. Grand challenges in chronic non-communicable diseases. *Nature* **450**: 494–6.

Dalal S, Beunza JJ, Volmink J, *et al.* 2011. Non-communicable diseases in sub-Saharan Africa: what we know now. *International Journal of Epidemiology* **40**: 885–901.

Deaton A. 1997. *The Analysis of Household Surveys: A Microeconomic Approach to Development Policy*. World Bank Publications: Washington, D.C.

Deb P, Munkin MK, Trivedi PK. 2006. Bayesian Analysis of the Two-Part Model with Endogeneity. Application to Health Care Expenditure. *Journal of Applied Econometrics* **21**: 1081–1099.

Donald SG, Green DA, Paarsch HJ. 2000. Differences in Wage Distributions between Canada and the United States: An Application of a Flexible Estimator of Distribution Functions in the Presence of Covariates. *The Review of Economic Studies* **67**: 609–33.

Dong H, Gbangou A, De Allegri M, Pokhrel S, Sauerborn R. 2008. The Differences in Characteristics between Health-Care Users and Non-Users. Implication for Introducing Community-Based Health Insurance in Burkina Faso. *The European Journal of Health Economics: HEPAC: Health Economics in Prevention and Care* **9**: 41–50.

Dor A, Gertler P, van der Gaag J. 1987. Non-price rationing and the choice of medical care providers in rural Cote d'Ivoire. *Journal of Health Economics* **6**: 291–304.

Dror DM, Jacquier C. 1999. Micro-Insurance. Extending Health Insurance to the Excluded. *International Social Security Review* **52**: 71–97.

Dror DM, van Putten-Rademaker O, Koren R. 2008. Cost of illness: evidence from a study in five resource-poor locations in India. *Indian Journal of Medical Research* **127**: 347–61.

Duan N, Manning WG, Morris CN, Newhouse JP. 1983. A Comparison of Alternative Models for the Demand for Medical Care. *Journal of Business & Economic Statistics* **1**: 115–26.

Efron B. 1988. Logistic Regression, Survival Analysis, and the Kaplan-Meier Curve. *Journal of the American Statistical Association* **83**: 414–25.

Elrayah H, Eltom M, Bedri A, Belal A, Rosling H, Östenson C-G. 2005. Economic burden on families of childhood type 1 diabetes in urban Sudan. *Diabetes Research and Clinical Practice* **70**: 159–65.

Elrayah-Eliadarous H, Yassin K, Eltom M, Abdelrahman S, Wahlström R, Ostenson C-G. 2010. Direct costs for care and glycaemic control in patients with type 2 diabetes in Sudan. *Experimental and Clinical Endocrinology & Diabetes* **118**: 220–5.

Engelgau M, Karan A, Mahal A. 2012. The Economic Impact of Non-Communicable Diseases on Households in India. *Globalization and Health* **8**: 9.

Faronbi JO, Oladepo RO, Faronbi GO, Olaogun AA. 2014. Blood Pressure Monitoring Practices and Health Seeking Behaviours among University Staff in Nigeria. *International Journal of Caring Sciences* **7**: 58–65.

Fosu GB. 1994. Childhood morbidity and health services utilization: cross-national comparisons of user-related factors from DHS data. *Social science & medicine* **38**: 1209–20.

Fox J. 2008. *Applied Regression Analysis and Generalized Linear Models*. SAGE Publications, Inc: Los Angeles.

Fu AZ, Chen L, Sullivan SD, Christiansen NP. 2011. Absenteeism and short-term disability associated with breast cancer. *Breast Cancer Research and Treatment* **130**: 235–42.

Gans J. 1988. *Evaluation of Data Collection and Coding for Medical Conditions in the National Medical Care Utilization and Expenditure Survey*. National Center for Health Statistics, Public Health Service: Washington, DC.

Gertler P, Gaag J van der. 1990. *The Willingness to Pay for Medical Care: Evidence from Two Developing Countries*. World Bank: Washington, D.C.

Getzen TE. 2000. Health care is an individual necessity and a national luxury: applying multilevel decision models to the analysis of health care expenditures. *Journal of Health Economics* **19**: 259–70.

Gilleskie DB, Mroz TA. 2004. A flexible approach for estimating the effects of covariates on health expenditures. *Journal of Health Economics* **23**: 391–418.

Gimenes HT, Zanetti ML, Haas VJ. 2009. Factors related to patient adherence to antidiabetic drug therapy. *Revista Latino-Americana De Enfermagem* **17**: 46–51.

Gnawali DP, Pokhrel S, Sié A, *et al.* 2009. The Effect of Community-Based Health Insurance on the Utilization of Modern Health Care Services. Evidence from Burkina Faso. *Health Policy* **90**: 214–22.

Goldman N, Lin I-F, Weinstein M, Lin Y-H. 2003. Evaluating the quality of self-reports of hypertension and diabetes. *Journal of Clinical Epidemiology* **56**: 148–54.

Goryakin Y, Suhrcke M. 2014. The prevalence and determinants of catastrophic health expenditures attributable to non-communicable diseases in low- and middle-income countries: a methodological commentary. *International Journal for Equity in Health* **13**: 107.

Gotsadze G, Bennett S, Ranson K, Gzirishvili D. 2005. Health care-seeking behaviour and out-of-pocket payments in Tbilisi, Georgia. *Health Policy and Planning* **20**: 232–42.

Gotsadze G, Zoidze A, Rukhadze N. 2009. Household catastrophic health expenditure: evidence from Georgia and its policy implications. *BMC Health Services Research* **9**: 69.

Gottret P, Schieber GJ, Waters HR. 2008. *Good Practices in Health Financing: Lessons from Reforms in Low- And Middle-Income Countries.* World Bank Publications: Washington, DC.

Gottret PE, Schieber G. 2006. *Health financing revisited: a practitioner's guide.* World Bank Publications: Washington, D.C.

Goudge J, Gilson L, Russell S, Gumede T, Mills A. 2009a. Affordability, availability and acceptability barriers to health care for the chronically ill: Longitudinal case studies from South Africa. *BMC Health Services Research* **9**: 75.

Goudge J, Gilson L, Russell S, Gumede T, Mills A. 2009b. The household costs of health care in rural South Africa with free public primary care and hospital exemptions for the poor. *Tropical Medicine and International Health* **14**: 458–467.

Grossman M. 1972. On the Concept of Health Capital and the Demand for Health. *The Journal of Political Economy* **80**: 233–55.

Guariguata L, de Beer I, Hough R, *et al.* 2012. Diabetes, HIV and other health determinants associated with absenteeism among formal sector workers in Namibia. *BMC Public Health* **12**: 44.

Guinhouya KM, Tall A, Kombate D, *et al.* 2010. Cost of stroke in Lomé (Togo).

Gustafsson-Wright E, Duynhouwer A, van der Gaag J, Schultsz C. 2012. The Burden of Chronic Disease on Households in Tanzania and Kenya: Evidence from the Health Insurance Fund Operational Research (A Study for USAID). USAID, Washington, DC.

Gwatkin DR, Guillot M, Heuveline P. 1999. The burden of disease among the global poor. *The Lancet* **354**: 586–9.

Hall V, Thomsen R, Henriksen O, Lohse N. 2011. Diabetes in Sub Saharan Africa 1999–2011: Epidemiology and public health implications. a systematic review. *BMC Public Health* **11**: 564.

Haque M, Emerson SH, Dennison CR, Navsa M, Levitt NS. 2005. Barriers to initiating insulin therapy in patients with type 2 diabetes mellitus in public-sector primary health care centres in Cape Town. *South African medical journal* **95**: 798–802.

Hardin JW, Hilbe J. 2007. *Generalized Linear Models and Extensions,*. Stata Press: College Station, Texas.

Hensher DA, Rose JM, Greene WH. 2005. *Applied choice analysis: a primer*. Cambridge University Press: Cambridge, UK.

Hidayat B, Thabrany H, Dong H, Sauerborn R. 2004. The Effects of Mandatory Health Insurance on Equity in Access to Outpatient Care in Indonesia. *Health Policy Planning* **19**: 322–35.

Hill SC, Miller GE. 2010. Health expenditure estimation and functional form: applications of the generalized gamma and extended estimating equations models. *Health economics* **19**: 608–27.

Hjelm K, Atwine F. 2011. Health-care seeking behaviour among persons with diabetes in Uganda: an interview study. *BMC International Health and Human Rights* **11**: 11–8.

Hjortsberg C. 2003. Why do the sick not utilise health care? The case of Zambia. *Health Economics* **12**: 755–770.

Huffman MD, Rao KD, Pichon-Riviere A, *et al.* 2011. A Cross-Sectional Study of the Microeconomic Impact of Cardiovascular Disease Hospitalization in Four Low- and Middle-Income Countries. *PLoS ONE* **6**: e20821.

Islam SMS, Lechner A, Ferrari U, *et al.* 2013. Social and economic impact of diabetics in Bangladesh: protocol for a case–control study. *BMC Public Health* **13**: 1217.

Iyalomhe GBS, Iyalomhe SI. 2010. Hypertension-related knowledge, attitudes and life-style practices among hypertensive patients in a sub-urban Nigerian community. *Journal of Public Health and Epidemiology* **2**: 71–7.

Jiang C, Ma J, Zhang X, Luo W. 2012. Measuring Financial Protection for Health in Families with Chronic Conditions in Rural China. *BMC Public Health* **12**: 988.

Kankeu HT, Saksena P, Xu K, Evans DB. 2013. The financial burden from non-communicable diseases in low- and middle-income countries: a literature review. *Health Research Policy and Systems* **11**: 1–12.

Kasl SV, Cobb S. 1966. Health behavior, illness behavior, and sick role behavior. I. Health and illness behavior. *Archives of environmental health* **12**: 246–66.

Kazaura MR, Kombe D, Yuma S, Mtiro H, Mlawa G. 2007. Health seeking behavior among cancer patients attending ocean road cancer institute, Tanzania. *East African Journal of Public Health* **4**: 19–22.

Kehoe R, Wu S-Y, Leske MC, Chylack LT. 1994. Comparing self-reported and physician-reported medical history. *American Journal of Epidemiology* **139**: 813–8.

Kemp JR, Mann G, Simwaka BN, Salaniponi FM, Squire SB. 2007. Can Malawi's poor afford free tuberculosis services? Patient and household costs associated with a tuberculosis diagnosis in Lilongwe. *Bulletin of the World Health Organization* **85**: 580–5.

Kengne AP, June-Rose Mchiza Z, Amoah AGB, Mbanya J-C. 2013. Cardiovascular Diseases and Diabetes as Economic and Developmental Challenges in Africa. *Progress in Cardiovascular Diseases* **56**: 302–13.

Khattab M, Khader YS, Al-Khawaldeh A, Ajlouni K. 2010. Factors associated with poor glycemic control among patients with type 2 diabetes. *Journal of Diabetes and Its Complications* 24: 84–9.

Kiawi E, Edwards R, Shu J, Unwin N, Kamadjeu R, Mbanya JC. 2006. Knowledge, attitudes, and behavior relating to diabetes and its main risk factors among urban residents in Cameroon: a qualitative survey. *Ethnicity & disease* 16: 503–9.

Kidanto HL, Kilewo CD, Moshiro C. 2002. Cancer of the cervix: knowledge and attitudes of female patients admitted at Muhimbili National Hospital, Dar es Salaam. *East African medical journal* 79: 467–75.

Kirigia JM, Sambo HB, Sambo LG, Barry SP. 2009. Economic burden of diabetes mellitus in the WHO African region. *BMC International Health and Human Rights* 9: 6.

Kohler H-P, Watkins SC, Behrman JR, *et al*. 2014. Cohort Profile: The Malawi Longitudinal Study of Families and Health (MLSFH). *International Journal of Epidemiology*.

Kolling M, Winkley K, von Deden M. 2010. 'For someone who's rich, it's not a problem'. Insights from Tanzania on diabetes health-seeking and medical pluralism among Dar es Salaam's urban poor. *Globalization and Health* 6: 8–16.

Kriegsman D, Penninx B, Van Eijk JT, Boeke AJ, Deeg DJ. 1996. Self-reports and general practitioner information on the presence of chronic diseases in community dwelling elderly. *Journal of Clinical Epidemiology* 49: 1407–17.

Kruk ME, Mbaruku G, Rockers PC, Galea S. 2008. User Fee Exemptions Are not Enough. Out-of-Pocket Payments for 'Free' Delivery Services in Rural Tanzania. *Tropical Medicine and International Health* 13: 1442–51.

Kwesiga B, Zikusooka CM, Ataguba JE. 2015. Assessing catastrophic and impoverishing effects of health care payments in Uganda. *BMC Health Services Research* 15: 30.

Lang K, Lines LM, Lee DW, Korn JR, Earle CC, Menzin J. 2009. Lifetime and treatment-phase costs associated with colorectal cancer: evidence from SEER-Medicare data. *Clinical Gastroenterology and Hepatology: The Official Clinical Practice Journal of the American Gastroenterological Association* 7: 198–204.

Langley G, Mary N. 2012. Health Seeking Behaviours of Women with Cervical Cancer. *Community Medicine & Health Education* 2: 1000170.

Lawson D. 2004. Determinants of Health Seeking Behaviour in Uganda – Is It Just Income and User Fees That Are Important? Development Economics and Public Policy Working Paper No. 30553. University of Manchester, Institute for Development Policy and Management (IDPM).

Le C, Zhankun S, Jun D, Keying Z. 2012. The Economic Burden of Hypertension in Rural South-West China. *Tropical Medicine and International Health*.

Lim SS, Gaziano TA, Gakidou E, *et al.* 2007. Prevention of cardiovascular disease in high-risk individuals in low-income and middle-income countries: health effects and costs. *The Lancet* 370: 2054–62.

Lopes Ibanez-Gonzalez D, Norris SA. 2013. Chronic Non-Communicable Disease and Healthcare Access in Middle-Aged and Older Women Living in Soweto, South Africa. *PLoS ONE* 8: e78800.

Lopez AD, Mathers CD, Ezzati M, Jamison DT, Murray CJ. 2006. Global and regional burden of disease and risk factors, 2001: systematic analysis of population health data. *The Lancet* 367: 1747–57.

MacKian S. 2003. A review of health seeking behaviour: problems and prospects. University of Manchester, Manchester, UK.

Maddala GS. 1983. *Limited-Dependent and Qualitative Variables in Econometrics*. Cambridge University Press: Cambridge, UK.

Makaula P, Bloch P, Banda HT, *et al.* 2012. Primary health care in rural Malawi – a qualitative assessment exploring the relevance of the community-directed interventions approach. *BMC Health Services Research* 12: 328.

Makinga PN, Beke A. 2013. A cross-sectional survey on the lifestyle and healthseeking behaviour of Basotho patients with diabetes. *South African Family Practice* 55: 190–5.

Makoka D, Kaluwa B, Kambewa P. 2007. Demand for Private Health Insurance Where Public Health Services are Free. The Case of Malawi. *Journal of Applied Sciences* 7: 3268–73.

Malik AM, Syed SIA. 2012. Socio-economic determinants of household out-of-pocket payments on healthcare in Pakistan. *International Journal for Equity in Health* 11: 1–7.

Mamo Y, Seid E, Adams S, Gardiner A, Parry E. 2007. A primary healthcare approach to the management of chronic disease in Ethiopia: an example for other countries. *Clinical Medicine (London, England)* 7: 228–31.

Manning WG. 1998. The logged dependent variable, heteroscedasticity, and the retransformation problem. *Journal of Health Economics* 17: 283–95.

Manning WG, Mullahy J. 2001. Estimating log models: to transform or not to transform? *Journal of Health Economics* 20: 461–94.

Maseko FC. 2010. Social health insurance in Malawi. Draft version 1.2. UNICEF, Malawi Country Office, Lilongwe.

Matsaganis M, Mitrakos T, Tsakloglou P. 2009. Modelling health expenditure at the household level in Greece. *The European Journal of Health Economics* 10: 329–36.

Mayosi BM, Flisher AJ, Lalloo UG, Sitas F, Tollman SM, Bradshaw D. 2009. The burden of non-communicable diseases in South Africa. *The Lancet* 374: 934–47.

Mazalale J, Muula A, Kambala C, *et al.* forthcoming. Determinants of non-facility based delivery in Malawi. *Tropical medicine and International Health*.

Mbanya JC, Motala AA, Sobngwi E, Assah FK, Enoru ST. 2010. Diabetes in sub-Saharan Africa. *The Lancet* 375: 2254–66.

Mbeh GN, Edwards R, Ngufor G, Assah F, Fezeu L, Mbanya J-C. 2010. Traditional healers and diabetes: results from a pilot project to train traditional healers to provide health education and appropriate health care practices for diabetes patients in Cameroon. *Global Health Promotion* 17: 17–26.

Mendis S. 2010. The policy agenda for prevention and control of non-communicable diseases. *British Medical Bulletin* 96: 23–43.

Mendis S, Fukino K, Cameron A, *et al.* 2007. The availability and affordability of selected essential medicines for chronic diseases in six low- and middle-income countries. *Bulletin of the World Health Organization* 85: 279–88.

Merkesdal S, Ruof J, Huelsemann JL, *et al.* 2005. Indirect cost assessment in patients with rheumatoid arthritis (RA): Comparison of data from the health economic patient questionnaire HEQ-RA and insurance claims data. *Arthritis Care & Research* 53: 234–40.

Ministry of Health Malawi. 2011. Malawi Health Sector Strategic Plan 2011–2016. Moving towards Equity and Quality. Ministry of Health (Malawi), Lilongwe.

Missions Atlas Project. 2011. REPUBLIC OF MALAWI | Snapshots Section. WorldMap, Texas.

Miszkurka M, Haddad S, Langlois É, Freeman E, Kouanda S, Zunzunegui M. 2012. Heavy burden of non-communicable diseases at early age and gender disparities in an adult population of Burkina Faso: world health survey. *BMC Public Health* 12: 24.

Mondal S, Kanjilal B, Peters David H, Lucas H. 2010. Catastrophic out-of-pocket payment for health care and its impact on households: Experience from West Bengal, India., Baltimore, MD.

Msyamboza KP, Dzamalala C, Mdokwe C, *et al.* 2012. Burden of cancer in Malawi; common types, incidence and trends: National population-based cancer registry. *BMC Research Notes* 5: 149–56.

Msyamboza KP, Ngwira B, Dzowela T, *et al.* 2011. The Burden of Selected Chronic Non-Communicable Diseases and their Risk Factors in Malawi. Nationwide STEPS Survey. *PloS one* 6: e20316.

Msyamboza KP, Savage EJ, Kazembe PN, *et al.* 2009. Community-Based Distribution of Sulfadoxine-Pyrimethamine for Intermittent Preventive Treatment of Malaria During Pregnancy Improved Coverage but Reduced Antenatal Attendance in Southern Malawi. *Tropical Medicina and International Health* 14: 183–9.

Mueller DH, Lungu D, Acharya A, Palmer N. 2011. Constraints to Implementing the Essential Health Package in Malawi. *PLoS ONE* 6: e20741.

Mugisha F, Kouyate B, Gbangou A, Sauerborn R. 2002. Examining out-of-pocket expenditure on health care in Nouna, Burkina Faso: implications for health policy. *Tropical Medicine & International Health* 7: 187–196.

Mukherjee K, Koul V. 2014. Economic burden of coronary heart disease on households in Jammu, India. *The Health Agenda* 2: 29–36.

Mukherjee S, Haddad S, Narayana D. 2011. Social class related inequalities in household health expenditure and economic burden: evidence from Kerala, south India. *International Journal for Equity in Health* 10: 1.

Muula AS, Maseko FC. 2006. How are health professionals earning their living in Malawi? *BMC Health Services Research* 6: 97.

Mwandira R. 2011. Examining equity in out-of-pocket expenditures and utilization of healthcare services in Malawi. Oregon State University, Corvallis, Oregon.

National Statistical Office (Malawi). 2005. Malawi Demographic and Health Survey 2004. National Statistical Office (Malawi), Zomba.

National Statistical Office (Malawi). 2008. 2008 Population and Housing Census. Preliminary Report. National Statistical Office (Malawi), Zomba.

National Statistical Office (Malawi). 2011. Malawi Demographic and Health Survey 2010. National Statistical Office (Malawi), Zomba.

National Statistical Office (Malawi). 2012a. Malawi – Third Integrated Household Survey, 2010/11. National Statistical Office (Malawi), Zomba.

National Statistical Office (Malawi). 2012b. Malawi 2008 census Info.

Nelder JA, Wedderburn RW. 1972. Generalized linear models. *Journal of the Royal Statistical Society* **135**: 370–84.

Nesbitt RC, Gabrysch S, Laub A, *et al.* 2014. Methods to measure potential spatial access to delivery care in low- and middle-income countries: a case study in rural Ghana. *International Journal of Health Geographics* **13**: 25.

Neuhann HF, Warter-Neuhann C, Lyaruu I, Msuya L. 2002. Diabetes care in Kilimanjaro region: clinical presentation and problems of patients of the diabetes clinic at the regional referral hospital-an inventory before structured intervention. *Diabetic medicine: a journal of the British Diabetic Association* **19**: 509–13.

Norfazilah A, Samuel A, Law P, *et al.* 2013. Illness perception among hypertensive patients in primary care centre UKMMC. *Malaysian Family Physicia* **8**: 19–25.

Nugent R, Feigl A. 2010. Where Have All the Donors Gone? Scarce Donor Funding for Non-Communicable Diseases. Center for Global Development, Washington D.C.

Nxumalo N, Alaba O, Harris B, Chersich M, Goudge J. 2011. Utilization of traditional healers in South Africa and costs to patients: findings from a national household survey. *Journal of public health policy* **32 Suppl 1**: S124–136.

Obi SN, Ozumba BC. 2008. Cervical cancer: Socioeconomic implications of management in a developing nation. *Journal of Obstetrics & Gynaecology* 28: 526–8.

Odili U, Okwuanasor E. 2012. ESTIMATING THE COST OF DIABETES HOSPITALIZATION IN A SECONDARY HEALTH CARE FACILITY. *Nigerian Journal of Pharmaceutical Sciences* 11: 49–57.

O'Donnell O, Doorslaer E van, Wagstaff A, Lindelow M. 2007. *Analyzing health equity using household survey data analyzing: A guide to techniques and their implementation.* the World Bank: Washington D. C.

OECD. 2007. Society at a Glance: OECD Social Indicators, 2006 edition. OECD, Paris.

Oke DA, Bandele EO. 2004. Misconceptions of hypertension. *Journal of the National Medical Association* 96: 1221–4.

Okunade AA, Suraratdecha C, Benson DA. 2010. Determinants of Thailand household healthcare expenditure: the relevance of permanent resources and other correlates. *Health Economics* 19: 365–376.

Onwujekwe OE, Uzochukwu BS, Obikeze EN, *et al.* 2010. Investigating determinants of out-of-pocket spending and strategies for coping with payments for healthcare in southeast Nigeria. *BMC Health Services Research* 10: 67.

Orem JN, Mugisha F, Okui AP, Musango L, Kirigia JM. 2013. Health care seeking patterns and determinants of out-of-pocket expenditure for Malaria for the children under-five in Uganda. *Malaria Journal* 12: 1–11.

Osamor PE. 2011. Health Care Seeking For Hypertension In South West Nigeria. *Medical Sociology online* 6: 54–69.

Osamor PE, Owumi BE. 2011. Factors Associated with Treatment Compliance in Hypertension in Southwest Nigeria. *Journal of Health, Population, and Nutrition* 29: 619–28.

Osborn CE. 2000. *Statistical Applications for Health Information Management.* Jones & Bartlett Learning: Burlington, MA.

Park RE. 1966. Estimation with Heteroscedastic Error Terms. *Econometrica* 34: 888.

Pepper DJ, Levitt NS, Cleary S, Burch VC. 2007. Hyperglycaemic emergency admissions to a secondary-level hospital – an unnecessary financial burden. *South African medical journal = Suid-Afrikaanse tydskrif vir geneeskunde* 97: 963–7.

Pestana JA, Steyn K, Leiman A, Hartzenberg GM. 1996. The direct and indirect costs of cardiovascular disease in South Africa in 1991. *South African Medical Journal* **86**: 679–84.

Petricca K, Mamo Y, Haileamlak A, Seid E, Parry E. 2009. BARRIERS TO EFFECTIVE FOLLOW-UP TREATMENT FOR RHEUMATIC HEART DISEASE IN JMMA, ETHIOPIA A GROUNDED THEORY ANALYSIS OF THE PATIENT EXPERIENCE. *Ethiop J Health Sci.* **19**: 39–44.

Phaswana-Mafuya N, Peltzer K, Chirinda W, *et al.* 2013. Self-reported prevalence of chronic non-communicable diseases and associated factors among older adults in South Africa. *Global Health Action* **6**.

Phillips PP, Phillips J, Aaron B. 2013. *Survey Basics: A Guide to Developing Surveys and Questionnaires*. American Society for Training and Development: U.S.

Phiri I, Masanjala W. 2012. Willingness to Pay for Micro Health Insurance in Malawi. In: Rösner H-J, Leppert G, Degens P, Ouedraogo L-M (eds). *Handbook of Micro Health Insurance in Africa*. 1st ed. Lit Verlag: Berlin, 285–308.

Pokhrel S, De Allegri M, Gbangou A, Sauerborn R. 2010. Illness reporting and demand for medical care in rural Burkina Faso. *Social Science & Medicine* **70**: 1693–700.

Preker AS, Carrin G, Dror D, Jakab M, Hsiao W, Arhin-Tenkorang D. 2004. Rich-Poor Differences in Health Care Financing. In: *Health Financing for Poor People – Resource Mobilization and Risk Sharing*. The World Bank: Washington, D.C., 3–52.

Rahman MM, Gilmour S, Saito E, Sultana P, Shibuya K. 2013. Health-Related Financial Catastrophe, Inequality and Chronic Illness in Bangladesh. *PLoS ONE* **8**: e56873.

Ramachandran A, Ramachandran S, Snehalatha C, *et al.* 2007. Increasing Expenditure on Health Care Incurred by Diabetic Subjects in a Developing Country: A study from India. *Diabetes Care* **30**: 252–6.

de Ramirez SS, Enquobahrie DA, Nyadzi G, *et al.* 2010. Prevalence and correlates of hypertension: a cross-sectional study among rural populations in sub-Saharan Africa. *Journal of Human Hypertension* **24**: 786–95.

Ramli A, Ahmad NS, Paraidathathu T. 2012. Medication adherence among hypertensive patients of primary health clinics in Malaysia. *Patient Preference and Adherence* **6**: 613–22.

Ravallion M, Chen S, Sangraula P. 2008. Dollar a Day Revisited. World Bank, Washington D.C.

Ridde V, Agier I, Jahn A, *et al.* 2014. The impact of user fee removal policies on household out-of-pocket spending: evidence against the inverse equity hypothesis from a population based study in Burkina Faso. *The European Journal of Health Economics* **16**: 1–10.

Ryan M, Bate A, Eastmond CJ, Ludbrook A. 2001. Use of Discrete Choice Experiments to Elicit Preferences. *Quality in Health Care* **10 Suppl 1**: i55–60.

van der Sande MA, Coleman RL, Schim van der Loeff MF, *et al.* 2001. A template for improved prevention and control of cardiovascular disease in sub-Saharan Africa. *Health policy and planning* **16**: 345–50.

Sauerborn R, Berman P, Nougtara A. 1996. Age Bias, but no Gender Bias, in the Intra-Household Resource Allocation for Health Care in Rural Burkina Faso. *Health Transition Review* **6**: 131–45.

Schmidt MI, Duncan BB, e Silva GA, *et al.* 2011. Chronic non-communicable diseases in Brazil: burden and current challenges. *The Lancet* **377**: 1949–61.

Schwarz J, Wyss K, Gulyamova ZM, Sharipov S. 2013. Out-of-pocket expenditures for primary health care in Tajikistan: a time-trend analysis. *BMC Health Services Research* **13**: 103.

Schwarzkopf L, Menn P, Leidl R, *et al.* 2012. Excess costs of dementia disorders and the role of age and gender – an analysis of German health and long-term care insurance claims data. *BMC Health Services Research* **12**: 165.

Seedat YK. 2000. Hypertension in developing nations in sub-Saharan Africa. *Journal of Human Hypertension* **14**: 739–47.

Shobhana R, Rama Rao P, Lavanya A, Williams R, Vijay V, Ramachandran A. 2000. Expenditure on health care incurred by diabetic subjects in a developing country – a study from southern India. *Diabetes Research and Clinical Practice* **48**: 37–42.

Soliman EZ, Juma H. 2008. Cardiac Disease Patterns in Northern Malawi: Epidemiologic Transition Perspective. *Journal of Epidemiology* **18**: 204–8.

Sridhar D, Morrison JS, Piot P. 2011. Getting the Politics Right for the September 2011 UN High Level Meeting on NCDs. Center for Strategic and International Studies, Washington, DC.

Steyn K, Levitt NS. 2006. Health Services Research in South Africa for Chronic Diseases of Lifestyle. In: *Chronic Diseases of Lifestyle in South Africa: 1995–2005*. South African Medical Research Council, Department of Medicine, University of Cape Town: Cape Town, South Africa.

Su TT, Flessa S. 2011. Determinants of household direct and indirect costs: an insight for health-seeking behaviour in Burkina Faso. *The European Journal of Health Economics*: 1–10.

Su TT, Kouyaté B, Flessa S. 2006a. Catastrophic Household Expenditure for Health Care in a Low-Income Society. A Study from Nouna District, Burkina Faso. *Bulletin of the World Health Organization* 84: 21–7.

Su TT, Pokhrel S, Gbangou A, Flessa S. 2006b. Determinants of household health expenditure on western institutional health care. *The European Journal of Health Economics* 7: 199–207.

Suhrcke M, Nugent RA, Stuckler D, Rocco L. 2006. Chronic Disease: An Economic Perspective. The Oxford Health Alliance, London.

Sun Q, Liu X, Meng Q, Tang S, Yu B, Tolhurst R. 2009. Evaluating the financial protection of patients with chronic disease by health insurance in rural China. *International Journal for Equity in Health* 8: 1–10.

Tagoe HA. 2013. Household burden of chronic diseases in Ghana. *Ghana Medical Journal* 46: 54–8.

Tharkar S, Devarajan A, Kumpatla S, Viswanathan V. 2010. The socioeconomics of diabetes from a developing country: A population based cost of illness study. *Diabetes Research and Clinical Practice* 89: 334–40.

Tipping G, Segall M. 1995. Health care seeking behaviour in developing countries. An annotated bibliography and literature review.

Train KE. 2009. *Discrete Choice Methods with Simulation*. Cambridge University Press: Cambridge, UK.

Trogdon JG, Hylands T. 2008. Nationally Representative Medical Costs of Diabetes by Time Since Diagnosis. *Diabetes Care* 31: 2307–11.

Tsang A, Von Korff M, Lee S, *et al.* 2008. Common chronic pain conditions in developed and developing countries: Gender and age differences and comorbidity with depression-anxiety disorders. *The Journal of Pain* 9: 883–91.

Uddin MJ, Alam N, Sarma H, Chowdhury MAH, Alam DS, Niessen L. 2014. Consequences of hypertension and chronic obstructive pulmonary disease, healthcare-seeking behaviors of patients, and responses of the health system: a population-based cross-sectional study in Bangladesh. *BMC Public Health* 14: 547.

United Nations Development Programme. 2013. The Rise of the South: Human Progress in a Diverse World. United Nations Development Programme, New York.

United Nations General Assembly. 2011. Political Declaration of the High-level Meeting of the General Assembly on the Prevention and Control of Non-communicable Diseases. United Nations, New York.

Unwin N, Setel P, Rashid S, *et al.* 2001. Noncommunicable diseases in sub-Saharan Africa: where do they feature in the health research agenda? *Bulletin of the World Health Organization* 79: 947–953.

Van Minh H, Xuan Tran B. 2012. Assessing the household financial burden associated with the chronic non-communicable diseases in a rural district of Vietnam. *Global Health Action* 5.

Van Minh H, Ng N, Juvekar S, *et al.* 2008. Self-Reported Prevalence of Chronic Diseases and Their Relation to Selected Sociodemographic Variables: A Study in INDEPTH Asian Sites, 2005. *Preventing Chronic Disease* 5: A86.

Wedderburn RWM. 1974. Quasi-likelihood functions, generalized linear models, and the Gauss—Newton method. *Biometrika* 61: 439–47.

WHO. 2006. Health Action in Crises. Malawi. World Health Organization, Geneva.

WHO. 2011a. From burden to 'best buys': Reducing the economic impact of NCDs in low- and middle-income countries. World Health Organization, Geneva.

WHO. 2011b. Uniting against NCDs, the Time to Act is Now: The Brazzaville Declaration on Noncommunicable Diseases Prevention and Control in the WHO African Region. World Health Organization Regional Office for Africa, Brazzaville.

World Bank. 2012. Household Questionnaire. Wolrd Bank, Washington D.C.

World Bank. 2014a. Out-of-pocket health expenditure (% of private expenditure on health).

World Bank. 2014b. World Development Indicators.

World Bank. 2014c. World Development Indicators: Poverty rates at international poverty lines.

World Bank. 2015. PPP conversion factor, GDP (LCU per international $).

World Health Organization. 1980. International Classification of Impairments, Disabilities and Handicaps. A manual of Classification Relating to the Consequences of Diseases. World Health Organization, Geneva.

World Health Organization. 2000. Prevention and control of noncommunicable diseases. World Health Organization, Geneva.

World Health Organization. 2003a. WHO Framework Convention on Tobacco Control. World Health Organization, Geneva.

World Health Organization. 2003b. Prevention and Control of Chronic Respiratory Diseases in Low and Middle-Income African Countries a Preliminary Report. World Health Organization, Geneva.

World Health Organization. 2004a. Global Strategy on Diet, Physical Activity and Health. World Health Organization, Geneva.

World Health Organization. 2004b. The world health report 2004 – changing history. World Health Organization, Geneva.

World Health Organization. 2005. Preventing Chronic Diseases: A Vital Investment. World Health Organization, Geneva.

World Health Organization. 2008a. The Global Burden of Disease: 2004 Update. World Health Organization, Geneva.

World Health Organization. 2008b. 2008–2013 Action plan for the global strategy for the prevention and control of noncommunicable diseases. World Health Organization, Geneva.

World Health Organization. 2008c. Projections of mortality and burden of disease, 2004–2030. World Health Organization, Geneva.

World Health Organization. 2008d. Prevention and Control of Noncommunicable Diseases: Implementation of the Global Strategy-report from the Secretory. World Health Organization, Geneva.

World Health Organization. 2010. Global Strategy to Reduce the Harmful Use of Alcohol. World Health Organization, Geneva.

World Health Organization. 2011a. Global Status Report on Noncommunicable Diseases 2010. World Health Organization, Geneva.

World Health Organization. 2011b. First global ministerial conference on healthy lifestyles and NCDs control. World Health Organization, Geneva.

World Health Organization. 2011c. Noncommunicable Diseases Country Profiles 2011. World Health Organization, Geneva.

World Health Organization. 2011d. From burden to 'best buys': Reducing the economic impact of NCDs in low- and middle-income countries. World Health Organization, Geneva.

World Health Organization. 2012. WHO Global Action Plan for the Prevention and Control of NCDs 2013–2020. World Health Organization, Geneva.

World Health Organization. 2014a. Non-communicable diseases.

World Health Organization. 2014b. Health financing: Health expenditure per capita Data by country.

World Health Organization Regional Office for Africa. 2000a. Noncommunicable Diseases: A Strategy for the African Region. World Health Organization Regional Office for Africa, Brazzaville.

World Health Organization Regional Office for Africa. 2000b. Oral Health in the African Region: A Regional Strategy 1999 – 2008. World Health Organization Regional Office for Africa, Brazzaville.

World Health Organization Regional Office for Africa. 2005. Cardiovascular Diseases in the African Region: Current Situation and Perspectives. World Health Organization Regional Office for Africa, Brazzaville.

World Health Organization Regional Office for Africa. 2006. Sickle-cell Disease in the African Region: Current Situation and the Way Forward. World Health Organization Regional Office for Africa, Brazzaville.

World Health Organization Regional Office for Africa. 2007. Diabetes Prevention and Control: A Strategy For the WHO African Region. World Health Organization Regional Office for Africa, Brazzaville.

World Health Organization Regional Office for Africa. 2008. Cancer Prevention and Control: A Strategy For the WHO African Region. World Health Organization Regional Office for Africa, Brazzaville.

World Health Organization Regional Office for Africa. 2011. Uniting against NCDs, the Time to Act is Now: The Brazzaville Declaration on Noncommunicable Diseases Prevention and Control in the WHO

African Region. World Health Organization Regional Office for Africa, Brazzaville.

Xu K, Evans DB, Kadama P, *et al.* 2006a. Understanding the impact of eliminating user fees: utilization and catastrophic health expenditures in Uganda. *Social Science & Medicine (1982)* **62**: 866–76.

Xu K, Evans DB, Kawabata K, Zeramdini R, Klavus J, Murray CJL. 2003. Household Catastrophic Health Expenditure. A Multicountry Analysis. *The Lancet* **362**: 111–7.

Xu K, James C, Carrin G, Muchiri S. 2006b. An Empirical Model of Access to Health Care, Health Care Expenditure and Impoverishment in Kenya. Learning from past Reforms and Lessons for the Future. World Health Oragnization, Geneva.

Yaffe R, Shapiro S, Fuchseberg RR, Rohde CA, Corpeno HC. 1978. Medical economics survey-methods study: cost-effectiveness of alternative survey strategies. *Medical Care* **16**: 641–59.

Yang G, Kong L, Zhao W, *et al.* 2008. Emergence of chronic non-communicable diseases in China. *The Lancet* **372**: 1697–705.

Yardim MS, Cilingiroglu N, Yardim N. 2014. Financial protection in health in Turkey: the effects of the Health Transformation Programme. *Health Policy and Planning* **29**: 177–92.

Yip WC, Wang H, Liu Y. 1998. Determinants of Patient Choice of Medical Provider: A Case Study in Rural China. *Health Policy and Planning* **13**: 311–22.

Zeidner M, Endler NS. 1995. *Handbook of Coping: Theory, Research, Applications.* John Wiley & Sons: New York.

Zere E, Walker O, Kirigia J, Zawaira F, Magombo F, Kataika E. 2010. Health financing in Malawi: Evidence from National Health Accounts. *BMC International Health and Human Rights* **10**: 27.

Zhang P, Zhang X, Brown J, *et al.* 2010. Global healthcare expenditure on diabetes for 2010 and 2030. *Diabetes Research and Clinical Practice* **87**: 293–301.

8. Appendices

8.1 Algorithm for grouping of reported non-communicable disorders and symptoms into illness categories

CNCD categories	Clinical and experiential expressions of chronic illness
Chronic respiratory conditions	Respiratory disorders & diseases *(asthma, emphysema, chronic obstructive lung disease, chronic bronchitis, chronic restrictive lung disease)*; Respiratory symptoms & impairments *(shortness of breath, dry cough, productive cough with colored sputum, wheezing, "recurrent gasping/loud breathing")*.
Chronic cardiovascular conditions	Cardiovascular disorders & diseases *(chronic hypertension, coronary heart disease, dysrhythmias, heart failure, chronic inflammatory heart disease, chronic sequelae of stroke)*; Cardiovascular symptoms & impairments *(right-sided chest pain/chest tightness, irregular/fast heartbeats, productive cough with clear sputum, edema, focal weakness of limbs, hemiparesis, dysarthria, "permanently loosing ones strength/speech")*.
Chronic neuropsychiatric conditions	Neuropsychiatric disorders & diseases *(depression, anxiety and panic disorders, stress disorders, dementia, schizophrenia, epilepsy, poliomyelitis, multiple sclerosis)*; Neuropsychiatric symptoms & impairments *(mood changes, longstanding anxiety or paranoia, memory loss, emotional stress, hallucinations, "being crazy", recurrent convulsions)*.
Malignant neoplastic conditions	Neoplastic disorders & diseases *(lung cancer, stomach/esophageal cancer, liver cancer, colorectal cancer, breast cancer, cervical/uterine cancer, prostate cancer, leukemia, lymphoma, brain tumor)*; Neoplastic symptoms & impairments *(indolent tumors/knots, night sweats, emaciation)*.
Chronic endocrine conditions	Endocrine disorders & diseases *(diabetes mellitus, thyroid disease)*; Endocrine symptoms & impairments *(high blood sugar, goiter)*.

CNCD categories	Clinical and experiential expressions of chronic illness
Chronic digestive conditions	Digestive disorders & diseases *(chronic reflux disease, chronic gastritis, peptic ulcer, chronic colitis, inflammatory bowel disease, rectal prolapse, hemorrhoids, intestinal hernia, hepatitis, chronic cholecystitis, gallstone disease, chronic pancreatitis)*; Digestive symptoms & impairments *(chronic diarrhea, recurrent heartburn, recurrent stomach pain, recurrent abdominal pain, jaundice, recurrent rectal bleed, dark stools, constipation, stool incontinence)*.
Chronic musculoskeletal conditions & chronic pain syndromes	Musculoskeletal disorders & diseases *(migraine, arthrosis, rheumatic arthritis, myalgia, paralysis)*; Musculoskeletal symptoms & impairments *(recurrent headaches, chronic joint pain/swelling, chronic back/neck pain, limb deformities, missing/stiff limbs, muscle soreness)*.
Chronic sense organ conditions	Sense organ disorders & diseases *(blindness, chronic conjunctivitis, trachoma, cataract, glaucoma, deafness, chronic sinusitis/rhinitis)*; Sense organ symptoms & impairments *(dryness of eyes, vision loss, hearing loss)*.
Chronic skin or oral conditions	Skin and oral disorders & diseases *(ectopic dermatitis, gangrene, guinea worm, ring worm, scabies)*; Skin symptoms & impairments *(recurrent itching/scaling of skin, recurrent rash, non-healing skin sores/ulcers)*.
Chronic genitourinary conditions	Genitourinary disorders & diseases *(kidney stone disease, pelvic inflammatory disease, chronic cystitis/prostatitis)*; Genitourinary symptoms & impairments *(frequent urination, urine incontinence, recurrent flank pain, painful menstruation, vaginal/penile discharge)*.

8.2 The questionnaire for CNCDs

In this section we would like to ask you about chronic illnesses. By chronic we mean any illness which you have that has lasted longer than three months or any illness that came up earlier in your life and has not disappeared until today.

1	Do you suffer from any of these chronic conditions (Please make sure to enter only chronic conditions): (If the respondent answer 'No' to any of these chronic conditions, please go to acute section)	Yes or No	If yes, for how many years have you had these chronic symptoms?
	Longstanding problems with lungs or breathing / Chronic respiratory infections or lung diseases (e.g. a. Asthma (wheezing attacks), b. Chronic bronchitis/emphysema/ COPD (chronic productive cough and wheezing), c. Pulmonary fibrosis/sarcoidosis (dry cough and shortness of breath))		
	Chronic high blood pressure / hypertension		
	Longstanding problem with the heart or blood circulation / cardiovascular diseases (e.g. a. Coronary artery disease (intermittent right-sided radiating chest pain), b. Dysrhythmias (irregular heart beats), c. Heart failure (oedema, shortness of breath), d. Inflammatory heart disease/rheumatic fever, e. Sequelae of brain stroke (focal weakness, abnormal speech))		
	Longstanding problems with the mood, chronic mental or psychiatric conditions (e.g. a. Depression, b. Longstanding anxiety/paranoia/PTSD, c. Dementia, Alzheimer d. Schizophrenia / psychotic disorder (often referred to as "being crazy"), e. Epilepsy / seizure disorder, f. Mental retardation / brain damage, cerebral palsy (meaning mentally handicapped since birth/childhood) g. Speech impediment)		
	Cancer, malignant tumor or neoplasms (e.g. Lung cancer, Stomach/oesophagous cancer, Liver cancer, Colorectal cancer, Breast cancer, Cervical/uterine cancer, Leukemia, Brain tumor, Lymphoma)		
	Raised blood sugar or Diabetes mellitus		
	Longstanding diseases of the stomach, bowel or the liver / chronic digestive diseases (e.g. a. Chronic diarrhoea/ malabsorption/ tropical sprue/ colitis/ Morbus Crohn, b. Heartburn / reflux disease, upset stomach/ gastritis / PUD, c. rectal prolapse / hemorrhoids(piles), d. Hepatitis / cirrhosis of liver / jaundice, e. gall stones / cholecystitis, f. Hernia)		

	Longstanding/chronic pains / aches (e.g. a. Recurrent headaches / migraine, b. Chronic back pain, c. joint pain / arthrosis, d. Arthritis / rheumatism, e. sickle cell)		
	Physical handicap, deformities or disabilities (longstanding problems with mobility, limb function (bones, legs, arms) (e.g. a. Difficulty walking / unable to walk, b. Missing / non-functional / stiff limbs)		
	Longstanding problems with the eyes, ears or nose: e.g. a. poor eyesight / blindness, b. Chronic conjunctivitis, c. Trachoma, e. Cataract, f. Poor hearing / deafness g. Chronic sinusitis		
	Longstanding problems with the skin / Dermatologic Diseases: (e.g. Ectopic Dermatitis, Gangrene, Guinea worm, Ringworm, Scabies)		
	Any other chronic diseases or other permanent diseases (lasting longer than the last three months) (If Yes, please go to question 2. If No, please go to question 3)		
2	Could you please describe the health problem(s) you had. (symptoms, syndromes). (please see symptom code and write down the code of symptom/symptoms answered by the respondent)		
	symptom or syndrome 1		
	symptom or syndrome 2		
	symptom or syndrome 3		
	symptom or syndrome 4		
3	Who did you consult for treatment for this/these chronic condition(s) during the last four weeks? *(1) Health care provider (western medicine); (2) Community health worker or community nurse; (3) Traditional healer or herbalist; (4) Myself/family members (self-treatment); (5) Did not seek treatment for this condition in the last four weeks* (If the answer is (1), (2), and (3), please go to questions 4, 5, 7; If the answer is (1) and (2), please go to questions 8, 9, 11, 17, 18; If the answer is (1), please go to questions 12, 13, 14, 15, 16; If the answer is (3), (4), and (5), please go directly to question 20)		

152

4	The treatment(s) for this/these chronic condition(s) in the last four weeks, was it a follow-up visit (e.g. for medication refill) or due to acute symptoms of the chronic condition or both? *(1) Follow-up visit/check-up; (2) Acute symptoms; (3) Both*		
5	During the last four weeks, were you supposed to take any drugs for this chronic condition? *(1) Yes; (2) No* (If Yes, please go to question 6; if No, please go to question 7)		
6	Did you run out of the required drugs during the last four weeks? *(1) Yes; (2) No*		
7	At what point since these chronic symptoms occurred did you decide to seek treatment from a health care provider during the last four weeks? *(1) Immediately; (2) Waited to see the severity of illness; (3) When it started affecting my day-to-day work; (4) When it started incapacitating me*		
8	Where specifically did you get your treatment during the last four weeks? *(1) General practitioner or clinic; (2) District hospital or other regional hospital; (3) Central hospital; (4) Mobile clinic; (5) Community health worker / village clinic; (6) Registered pharmacies for consultation and drugs; (8) Health centre; (99) Other*		
9	What is the name of the facility? (please see facility code and write down the code of facility answered by the respondent) (If Other, please go to question 10)		
10	If other facility, please write the name of the facility (including the village/city)		
11	What was the most important reason for choice of this provider? (1) Referral; (2) Close proximity or easy to reach; (3) Better services; (4) Lower cost of service; (5) Shorter waiting time; (6) I have personal relations; (7) I received financial or in-kind incentives to go there; (8) Provider is contracted by medical insurance scheme; (9) I had no other option		
12	If you went to a health facility, was this health facility private, CHAM or Public? (1) Private; (2) CHAM; (3) Public; (98) Do not know		

13	If you went to a health facility, what was your main means of transport during the last four weeks? (1) Walking; (2) Public transport; (3) Hire taxi; (4) Cart; (5) Bicycle; (6) Motorbike; (7) Car; (8) By ambulance; (99) Other		
14	How many hours did it take you to get to the facility?		
15	How many hours did you have to wait to be seen by the health personnel during the last four weeks? (beginning from the time you entered the facility)		
16	During the last four weeks, have you had to stay in hospital for this/these chronic condition(s)? (1) Yes; (2) No		
17	If yes, how many nights did you sleep in the facility in total?		
18	Overall, how satisfied were you with the services you received in the facility used? (1) very satisfied; (2) somewhat satisfied; (3) neither satisfied nor unsatisfied; (4) somewhat unsatisfied; (5) very unsatisfied		
19	Would you recommend the facility to family or friends? (1) Yes; (2) No		
20	Which reason best explains why you did not seek treatment at a health care provider (western medicine)? (1) Expensive medical treatment; (2) Minor complaints that don't call for professional assistance; (3) Poor public health services; (4) Long wait to meet doctor; (5) No transport available; (6) Could not get time because of work or had other commitments; (7) Went to the facility but could not get public health care; (8) Family (spouse, in-laws) decided otherwise; (99) Other		
21	Were any drugs given directly to you for free for this/these chronic condition(s) by the health staff treating you during the last four weeks? (1) Yes; (2) No		
22	Were any drugs prescribed for this/these chronic condition(s) by health staff to be obtained during the last four weeks? (inside or outside the facility) (1) Yes; (2) No (If Yes, please go to question 23; if Yes, please go to question 24)		

23	Did you obtain all prescribed medicines? (1) Yes; (2) No (If Yes, please go to question 26; if No, please go to question 24 and 25)		
24	How often did you not obtain the prescribed medicine during the last four weeks? (1) Never obtained the prescribed medicine; (2) Rarely obtained the prescribed medicine; (3) Sometimes obtained the prescribed medicine; (4) Often obtained the prescribed medicine		
25	If prescribed drugs were not obtained, which reasons best explain why you did not obtain them? (1) Forgot to buy; (2) Drugs not available; (3) Used home made medicine instead; (4) Too expensive; (5) Did not have money; (6) Do not trust these drugs; (7) Felt no need to do so; (8) Negative side-effects of drugs; (99) Other		
26	How much did you have to pay for the following treatment items in relation to this/these chronic condition in the last four weeks?		
	All consultation and treatment costs for this/these condition(s), including: laboratory tests (X-rays etc.), drugs (tablets, injections, infusions, topical preparations etc.), medical devices (crutches, glasses, etc.), as well as informal fees.		
	Costs for traditional healers, herbalists, faith healers		
	Transportation (incl. Fuel)		
27	How did you pay for all the health care expenditure that you incurred for this/these chronic condition(s) in the last four weeks? (1) I did not have to pay (services were for free); (2) Another institution paid all for me (e.g. insurer, NGO, employer); (3) Another institution paid something for me (e.g. insurer, NGO, employer) and I paid the rest out-of-pocket; (4) I paid everything out-of-pocket; (5) I was supposed to pay out of pocket but did not have the money at that moment and I am still expected to pay (If the answer is (2) or (3), please go to question; If the answer is (3), (4), or (5), please go to question 29;		

28	If another institution paid something/all for your treatment, what institution was it? (1) Employer; (2) Insurer; (3) NGO (incl. pre-paid voucher or cash incentives); (4) Government programme (incl. pre-paid voucher or cash incentives); (5) Churches/mosques etc.; (99) Other		
29	From which source (s) did you raise money to pay for these out-of-pocket payments?		
	Cash at home (1) Yes; (2) No		
	Used SACCO savings (1) Yes; (2) No		
	Used other bank savings (1) Yes; (2) No		
	Used SACCO loans (1) Yes; (2) No		
	Used other bank loans (1) Yes; (2) No		
	Rotating savings and credit club (ROSCA) (1) Yes; (2) No		
	Borrowed money from money lender (1) Yes; (2) No		
	Borrowed money from friends/relatives (1) Yes; (2) No		
	Assistance from friends and relatives (I don't have to pay it back) (1) Yes; (2) No		
	Sold an asset (1) Yes; (2) No		
	National remittances (member of family who is not living in household for more than three months) (1) Yes; (2) No		
	International remittances (1) Yes; (2) No		
	Other (1) Yes; (2) No		

30	Did your chronic conditions hinder you from carrying out routine activities? (1) Yes; (2) No (If Yes, please go to question 31 and 32; if No, please go to question 33)		
31	How many days could you not carry out routine activities during the last four weeks due to these chronic conditions?		
32	How many people (adults) took care of you throughout the course of treatment for these chronic conditions, i.e., from when you were unable to carry out routine activities until you got better?		
33	Did you have to pay the people who took care of you throughout the course of treatment for these chronic conditions? (1) Yes; (2) No		
34	How much did you pay them to take care of you?		
35	How many of these people who took care of you are female? (If no less than 1 person took care of you, please go to question 36)		
36	Did your chronic conditions prevent people that took care of you from working? (1) Yes; (2) No		

Symptom code	

Symptom code

General Symptoms
1. Dehydration / Fluid loss
2. Fainting / Passing out
3. Fatigue / Lethargy
4. Fever / Chills
5. Loss of appetite / Unable to breast feed
6. Night sweats
7. Swelling feet / legs / body
8. Weight loss

Skin:
11. Boils / Abscess on skin
12. Itching
13. Jaundice / Yellow eyes
14. Pallor
15. Skin rash / blisters / localized swelling
16. Skin sore / Ulcer / Gangrene

Head & Face:
21. Congested / runny nose
22. Ear pain
23. Eye pain / tearing / redness
24. Facial rash / Swelling of face
25. Headache
26. Hearing loss
27. Jaw-lock
28. Nose bleeding
29. Sore Throat / Difficulties swallowing
30. Toothache / Sore mouth
31. Vision loss

Mental Status:
41. Abnormal behaviour / speech / cognition
42. Anxiety
43. Confusion
44. Convulsions
45. Dizziness / Spinning sensation
46. Insomnia / Sleeplessness
47. Loss of consciousness
48. Sadness
49. Suicidal ideation
50. Addiction (alcohol, drugs, tobacco)

Neck & Back:
51. Back / neck pain
52. Neck swelling
53. Stiff Neck

Chest & Respiration:
61. Cough (dry / with sputum / with blood)
62. Chest pain / tightness / pressure
63. Difficulty breathing / Shortness of breath / Wheezing
64. Rapid Heartbeat / palpitations

Abdomen & Digestion:
71. Abdominal / Pelvic / Flank pain or cramping
72. Anal / rectal pain
73. Blood in vomit / stool / urine
74. Constipation
75. Diarrhoea
76. Nausea / vomiting
77. Stomach pain / Heartburn

Urinary Tract & Genitals:
81. Abnormal vaginal bleeding
82. Frequent urination
83. Menstrual cramps / pain
84. Painful / burning urination / Dark urine
85. Urine / Stool incontinence
86. Vaginal / Penile discharge / sores / ulcers
87. Vaginal bleeding / Painful menstruation

Muscles, Bones & Joints:
91. Joint pain / Bone pain
92. Joint swelling
93. Muscle soreness / pain (myalgia)
94. Paralysis / Palsy

Pregnancy / Delivery / Newborn:
96. Prolonged labour
97. Prolonged bleeding after delivery / postnatal hemorrhage
98. Pain / Vaginal bleeding during pregnancy

Facility code	
1. Bilal Dispensary (Chiradzulu)	36. St Joseph Health Centre (Thyolo), CHAM
2. Chipho Health Centre (Chiradzulu), CHAM	37. Thekerani Health Centre (Thyolo)
3. Chiradzulu District Hospital (Chiradzulu)	38. Thomas Health Centre (Thyolo), CHAM
4. Chitera Health Centre (Chiradzulu)	39. Thyolo District Hospital (Thyolo)
5. Magomero Health Centre (Chiradzulu), CHAM	40. Zoa Health Centre (Thyolo)
6. Mauwa Health Centre (Chiradzulu)	41. Mlambe Hospital (Blantyre), CHAM
7. Mbulumbuzi Health Centre (Chiradzulu)	42. Queen Elizabeth Central Hospital (Blantyre)
8. Milepa Health Centre (Chiradzulu)	43. Mulanje Mission Hospital (Mulanje), CHAM
9. Namadzi Health Centre (Chiradzulu)	44. Pirimiti Community Hospital (Zomba), CHAM
10. Namitambo Health Centre (Chiradzulu)	45. St Lukes Hospital (Zomba), CHAM
11. Ndunde Health Centre (Chiradzulu)	46. Zomba Central Hospital (Zomba)
12. Nkalo Health Centre (Chiradzulu)	47. Bondo Health Centre (Mulanje)
13. PIM Health Centre (Chiradzulu), CHAM	48. Chambe Health Centre (Mulanje)
14. St Joseph Hospital (Chiradzulu), CHAM	49. Chinyama Health Centre (Mulanje)
15. Bvumbwe BLM Clinic (Thyolo)	50. Chisitu Health Centre (Mulanje)
16. Bvumbwe Makungwa Maternity (Thyolo)	51. Chonde Health Centre (Mulanje)
17. Bvumbwe Research Health Centre (Thyolo)	52. Dzenje (Maternity) (Mulanje)
18. Changata Health Centre (Thyolo)	53. Kambenje Health Centre (Mulanje)
19. Chimaliro Health Centre (Thyolo)	54. Mbiza Health Centre (Mulanje)
20. Chimvu Maternity (Thyolo)	55. Milonde Health Centre (Mulanje)
21. Chingadzi Community Hospital (Thyolo), CHAM	56. Mimosa Dispensary (Mulanje)
22. Gombe Maternity (Thyolo)	57. Mpala Health Centre (Mulanje)
23. Hellena Oakley Health Centre (Mtambanyama) (Thyolo), CHAM	58. Mulanje BLM Clinic (Mulanje)
24. Khonjeni Health Centre (Thyolo)	59. Mulanje District Hospital (Mulanje)
25. Makapwa Health Centre (Thyolo), CHAM	60. Mulanje Mission Hospital (Mulanje)
26. Malamulo Hospital (Thyolo), CHAM	61. Mulomba Health Centre (Mulanje)
27. Mangunda Clinic (Maternity) (Thyolo)	62. Muloza Health Centre (Mulanje)
28. Mapanga Clinic (Thyolo)	63. Namasalima Health Centre (Mulanje)
29. Mayaka Health Centre (Thyolo), CHAM	64. Namphungo Health Centre (Mulanje)
30. Mbalanguzi Dispensary (Thyolo), CHAM	65. Namulenga Health Centre (Mulanje)
31. Mikolongwe Health Centre (Thyolo)	66. Naphimba Health Centre (Mulanje)
32. Mitengo Health Centre (Thyolo)	67. Thembe Health Centre (Mulanje)
33. Molere Health Centre (Thyolo)	68. Thuchila Health Centre (Mulanje)
34. Nkhataombere Maternity (Thyolo)	99. Other facility (please specify)
35. Nsabwe Dispensary (Thyolo)	

8.3 Consent form

Respondent's name	
Respondent's MUSCCO ID	
Respondent's research ID	
Respondent's household ID	
Date of the interview	
Interviewer's name	

Before we begin, I would like to explain to you the aim of my visit, to clarify the use of the information that you will share with me, and to collect your explicit informed consent to proceed with the interview.

My name is ... and I am an interviewer working for REACH Trust, a Malawian institution committed to research in equity and community health. In collaboration with colleagues from the University of Heidelberg in Germany, we are conducting a study to assess people's access to health care services in your region, both before and after the introduction of the micro health insurance managed by MUSCCO. The information you will share with us will help us inform policy making with regard to the improvement of services related to the provision of health care in your region.

We would like to ask you and other members of your family information about your household, your illness profile in the last few weeks, and your access to health care services. We will ask you a lot of information that you will consider personal and we will store this information in a database.

Our research team from the University of Heidelberg and from REACH Trust, however, commits itself to treat this information with the highest level of confidentiality possible. I will not discuss the contents of this interview with anyone else, neither within nor beyond my study team. All the information that you will share with me will be entered in a database not containing your name, but simply an identification code to track households and individuals within households. The database will remain exclusive property of the research team and will only be used to compile analysis on access to care and relevant issues. Under no circumstances, the database as a whole or any subportion will be shared with other institutions.

If you are a MUSCCO member, we kindly ask you for permission to link the information that you will share with us through means of this interview

160

with information on your loan history kept in the MUSCCO records. Again, this match will be done anonymously, using your MUSCCO identification code, so that the researchers in charge of this activity will never be able to identify you as a person.

If you have children below 14, please answer the questions for your children. If you have children between 14 to 18, children can answer the questions themselves if you agree them to do so and you need another signature of your decision.

Participation in this study is voluntary. You have the right to refuse the interview or to refuse to answer any specific question. Participation in the study does not entail any direct risk or any direct benefit. You will incur into no consequences should you decide not to participate in this interview.

You can withdraw your participation at any point in time, without any need to motivate your decision. Withdrawal from the study will not yield any consequence for you, for your membership in MUSCCO and in its insurance program, nor for the medical care you will receive at any of the local facilities.

Should you decide to withdraw from the study, you can also ask to destroy all the information so far collected on you. Upon withdrawal from the study, you can also indicate whether you allow us to use the information collected so far or not. At any future point in time, you are free to change your mind and contact the person in charge of data collection to express your wish.

If you have any specific question, please feel free to ask me. I will be happy to answer you.

Thank you in advance for your cooperation.

I (interviewer's name) certify that I have correctly translated all of the above text to the respondent, that I have answered all relevant questions, and that he/she has understood the content of the information I shared with him.

Interviewer's signature ....

I declare that I have been verbally informed of all the details of the study.

I declare that I was given the opportunity to ask questions and that all my questions received satisfactory answers.

I declare that it was clarified to me and that I agree with the fact that the information collected from me for this study will be stored, used, and potentially forwarded to others anonymously. Third parties will at no point in time have access to my personal information. My name will not be disclosed during the process of publishing the results of the study.

I reserve the right to withdraw from the study and/or to withdraw the material collected from me at any point in time.

Respondent's signature ....

I declare that as parents between 14 to 18, I would like my children to answer all the questions. Once I see some problems of my children answering the questions, I reserve the right to stop my children doing so and let myself answer the questions for them.

Respondent's signature ....

Challenges in Public Health

Im Zeitalter der Globalisierung lässt sich *Public Health* nicht mehr allein innerhalb von nationalen Grenzen betreiben: Pandemien, abnehmende Trinkwasservorräte und steigender Tabakkonsum sind nur einige Beispiele für eine Vielzahl von neuen Herausforderungen, die einen weiter reichenden, internationalen Blick erfordern. Zusätzlich trägt eine einseitig an Wirtschaftsinteressen orientierte Globalisierung zu der weltweit zunehmenden gesundheitlichen Ungleichheit bei. Die Globalisierung eröffnet andererseits aber neue Wege, auch über Staatsgrenzen und große Entfernungen hinweg Wissen und Erfahrungen auszutauschen und gemeinschaftlich zu handeln. Kernpunkte für *Public Health* sind dabei die international vergleichende Analyse von Gesundheitsproblemen und möglichen Lösungsansätzen sowie die wissenschaftlich basierte und gerechte Ausgestaltung von Gesundheitssystemen. Hierzu möchte die Buchreihe *Challenges in Public Health* einen Beitrag leisten.

In times of globalisation, Public Health can no longer be practiced within national borders alone. Pandemics, diminishing drinking water supplies and increasing tobacco consumption are examples of the many new challenges that require a cross-border, international approach. In addition, a globalisation that is narrowly focused on economic interests contributes to growing health inequalities worldwide. At the same time, globalisation offers new opportunities to exchange knowledge and experiences and to collaborate across national borders. Key issues for Public Health are an international comparison of health problems and of possible strategies to solve them, as well as an evidence-based and equitable development of health systems. The book series *Challenges in Public Health* aims to contribute to this endeavour.

Medizin in Entwicklungsländern

Herausgegeben von Prof. Hans Jochen Diesfeld

Band 37 Andrea Materlik: Medizinisch-anthropologische Aspekte von Lepra im Amazonas und ihre Bedeutung für die Gesundheitserziehung. 1994.

Band 38 Oliver Razum: Improving Service Quality through Action Research, as applied in the Expanded Programme on Immunization (EPI). 1994.

Band 39 Ulrich Schramm: Einflußfaktoren auf die Akzeptanz von baulichen Anlagen der ländlichen Gesundheitseinheiten in Ägypten. Fallstudie am Beispiel der staatlichen Einheit in Zebeda unter Verwendung der Post-Occupancy Evaluation. 1995.

Band 40 Rainer Sauerborn / Adrien Nougtara / Hans Jochen Diesfeld (Eds.): Recherche sur les systèmes de santé: Le cas de la zone médicale de Solenzo, Burkina Faso. Auteurs: Rainer Sauerborn, Adrien Nougtara, Hans Jochen Diesfeld, Gaston Sorgho, Joseph Bidiga, Lougousse Tiébélessé, Eric Latimer, Roberto Sallier de La Tour, Uwe Brinkmann, Don Shepard. 1995.

Band 41 Rainer Sauerborn / Adrien Nougtara / Hans Jochen Diesfeld (Eds.): Les Côuts Economiques de la Maladie pour les Ménages au Milieu Rural du Burkina Faso. Avec des contributions de Rainer Sauerborn, Adrien Nougtara, Maurice Hien, Issouf Ibrango, Matthias Borchert, Justus Benzler, Eberhard Koob, Hans Jochen Diesfeld. 1996.

Band 42 Erhard Hinz: Helminthiasen des Menschen in Thailand. 1996.

Band 43 Matthias Perleth: Historical Aspects of American Trypanosomiasis (Chagas' Disease). 1997.

Band 44 Christiane Fischer: Über die Effektivität der Dorfgesundheitsarbeiterinnen innerhalb der Nichtregierungsorganisation ACCORD in Tamil Nadu/Südindien. Aktionsforschung im Rahmen der Gesundheitssystemforschung. 1998.

Band 45 Maureen Dar Iang: Assessment of antenatal and obstetric care services in a rural district of Nepal. 1999.

Band 46 Julia Katzan: sòi mendan – Die Sache mit dem Wasser... Eine medizinethnologische Untersuchung zum Zusammenhang von Wasser und Krankheit aus indigener Sicht. 2001.

Band 47 Catharina Will: Malaria-Selbstmedikation mit Chloroquin in einem hyperendemischen Gebiet (Mali). 2001.

Band 48 Ansgar Gerhardus: Entscheidungsprozesse im Gesundheitssektor. Der Beitrag der Theorie der politischen Ökonomie. 2001.

Band 49 Sylvie Schuster: Der Schwangerschaftsabbruch im Grasland Kameruns. Medizin, Kultur und Praxis. 2004.

Band 50 Sascha Klotzbücher: Das ländliche Gesundheitswesen der VR China. Strukturen – Akteure – Dynamik. 2006.

Challenges in Public Health

Editor: Prof. Dr. Oliver Razum

Band 51 Ulrich Ronellenfitsch: Cardiovascular Mortality among Ethnic German Immigrants from the Former Soviet Union. 2007.

Band 52 Manuela De Allegri: To Enrol or not to Enrol in Community Health Insurance. Case Study from Burkina Faso. 2007.

Band 53 Catherine Kyobutungi: Ethnic German Immigrants from the Former Soviet Union: Mortality from External Causes and Cancers. 2008.

Band 54 Maren Bredehorst: Information Systems for the Rehabilitation of Landmine Survivors. 2007.

Band 55 Sven Voigtländer / Gabriele Berg-Beckhoff / Oliver Razum: Gesundheitliche Ungleichheit. Der Beitrag kontextueller Merkmale. 2008.

Band 56 Oliver Razum / Jürgen Breckenkamp / Pitt Reitmaier (Hrsg.): Kindergesundheit in Entwicklungsländern. 2008.

Band 57 Steffen Fleßa: Costing of Health Care Services in Developing Countries. A Prerequisite for Affordability, Sustainability and Efficiency. 2009.

Band 58 Patrick Brzoska / Oliver Razum: Validity Issues in Quantitative Migrant Health Research. The Example of Illness Perceptions. 2010.

Band 59 Oliver Razum / Anna Reeske / Jacob Spallek (Hrsg.): Gesundheit von Schwangeren und Säuglingen mit Migrationshintergrund. 2011.

Band 60 Olaf Müller: Malaria in Africa. Challenges for Control and Elimination in the 21st Century. 2011.

Band 61 Walter Bruchhausen / Helmut Görgen / Oliver Razum (Hrsg.): Entwicklungsziel Gesundheit. Zeitzeugen der Entwicklungszusammenarbeit blicken zurück. 2011.

Band 62 Oliver Razum / Jacob Spallek / Anna Reeske / Melina Arnold (eds.): Migration-sensitive Cancer Registration in Europe. Challenges and Potentials. 2011.

Band 63 Martin Kohls: Demographie von Migranten in Deutschland. 2012.

Band 64 Patrick Brzoska: Psychometrically Relevant Differences between Source and Migrant Populations. 2014.

Band 65 Pauline Grys: Schistosomiasis Control in China. Diagnostics and Control Strategies Leading to Success. 2016.

Band 66 Qun Wang: Health Seeking Behavior and Out-of-pocket Expenditure on Chronic Noncommunicable Diseases in Sub-Saharan Africa. The Case of Rural Malawi. 2018.

www.peterlang.com